A WEEK BY WEEK GUIDE TO YOUR
PREGNANCY

NINA GRUNFELD

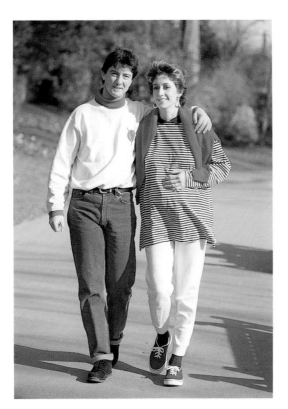

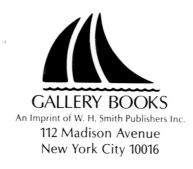

GALLERY BOOKS

An Imprint of W. H. Smith Publishers Inc.
112 Madison Avenue
New York City 10016

Contents

To my mother

First published in 1988 by
Conran Octopus Limited
37 Shelton Street
London WC2H 9HN

This edition published
in 1989 by Gallery Books,
an imprint of W.H. Smith Publishers Inc.,
112 Madison Avenue, New York, New York 10016,
in association with Conran Octopus Limited

Text copyright © 1988, 1989 Nina Grunfeld
Artwork copyright © 1988. 1989 Conran Octopus Limited

Reprinted 1990 . 1991

ISBN 0-8317-7134-8
Typeset by Tradespools Limited
Printed and bound in Hong Kong

Introduction

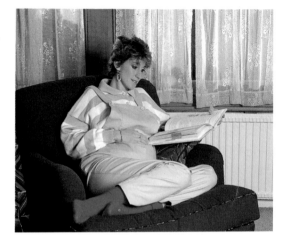

This book is a week-by-week guide to what is happening to you and your baby throughout your pregnancy.

On the left-hand pages, "You and Your Developing Baby" describes the physical and emotional changes you experience and the detailed development of your baby. You will find this a useful guideline although, of course, every woman – and every pregnancy – is different so you may feel that what appears under "You" in Week 7, for example, fits your Week 9 better. In the same way, the weights given for the baby – particularly in the later weeks – can only be an average guide.

You might like to use the diary space on the left-hand pages to write down important appointments and keep a note of your feelings; this will make an interesting record of your pregnancy for later on. We have given important reminders in the relevant weeks under "Don't forget": for example, your first prenatal visit, making a dental appointment or noting down when you first feel your baby kick.

The right-hand pages for each week feature particular aspects of pregnancy in some detail, from the first doctor's visit to shopping for the layette and baby equipment, as well as advice to expectant fathers and how to prepare yourselves for the birth itself. Some of these features, for example the amniocentesis test and ultrasound scan, are particularly relevant to a certain week while others may vary and many are relevant throughout your pregnancy. Cross-references are included wherever necessary to help you find all the information you want and there is also a full index at the back of the book.

Since medically your pregnancy is dated from the first day of your last period, and not from the time of conception, you may not know you are expecting a baby until you are at least "five weeks pregnant" – which is actually about two to three weeks after conception, and around the time of your first missed period.

The first few weeks of this book will, in effect, have already happened! You will find them interesting to read before you start following the weeks of the guide. The weeks of your pregnancy may not run from Monday to Sunday as in this book. If, for example, the first day of your last period was a Wednesday, your pregnancy weeks will run from Wednesday to Tuesday. Use the week closest to your own timing.

Each week, fill in the Month and Dates at the top of the page for that particular week – for example, November 24th–30th – so that you can use the diary space for specific appointments.

Throughout the diary your baby is referred to as "he", not because of any bias but just to differentiate you, the mother, from your baby. The term "partner" has been chosen to cover the expectant father, no matter what his status.

During pregnancy you will come across lots of new words and terms, especially medical ones. There is a short glossary of the more important of these at the back of the book. Never allow yourself to be confused by these – always ask the doctor what they mean if you do not understand the terms they are using.

There is also a list of useful addresses at the end of the book. Refer to the groups or associations if you would like more information about any particular topic. For example, if you are expecting twins you may like to know more than can be covered in this book and would find it helpful to contact the Mothers of Twins Clubs.

The forty weeks of pregnancy are conventionally divided into three terms, known medically as "trimesters". Many women find that, physically and emotionally, their pregnancy falls into three parts too. Forty weeks can seem a long time and you may find it helpful to have it broken down in some way. We have used colored bands to differentiate these three terms throughout the book and to help you relate the forty weeks to the actual months of your pregnancy.

A note about the author
When she was about fifteen weeks pregnant, Nina Grunfeld decided to write a book about what happens to mothers and their babies, week by week, during pregnancy. She was by then feeling well, happy and excited about her baby and wanted to convey the emotional ups and downs, the pleasures and concerns of pregnancy.

In Week 40 this book was finished and her first child, Michael, was born.

Nina Grunfeld is 34 years old, and this is her sixth book.

Week 1

MON

TUES

WED

THURS

FRI

SAT

SUN

Notes

PREGNANCY TESTS

The first, and most reliable, sign of your pregnancy will be a missed period. A less reliable sign will be that you just "feel pregnant". To test whether or not you are pregnant, you can buy a home testing kit from your pharmacist or you can have a pregnancy test done at your doctor's or your family planning clinic.

The most common pregnancy tests work by detecting a particular hormone in your urine. There is a more concentrated amount of this pregnancy hormone in the first urine you pass in the day, so you need to collect an early-morning sample in a clean, soap-free container. This hormone will show up about four weeks after conception, that is two weeks after the first day of your missed period. If you can't wait, a blood test can tell if you are pregnant before you have missed a period.

Follow the instructions with a kit very carefully. Positive results from a urine test are 99 per cent reliable. If your test is negative then it could be that there isn't yet enough pregnancy hormone to show up in a test. If your period doesn't start, have another test in a week's time.

This is one of several kinds of home testing kit. They all vary slightly so follow the instructions on the package.

Now you're pregnant

Congratulations on your pregnancy!

You may be one of the lucky ones who find the next forty or so weeks just fly by. Or you may feel pregnancy is a long process during which your body takes over your life. Every woman is different – and every pregnancy is too. Your feelings about pregnancy and parenthood will no doubt change constantly during the course of your pregnancy. Having a baby is rather like going on a blind date – but the build-up is forty weeks and the consequences lifelong!

The first fourteen weeks of your pregnancy may well be the hardest, so if you are feeling below par in the initial stages, take heart that things will improve. During early pregnancy, despite the excitement of expecting a baby, you may well feel exhausted and possibly sick. Even if you've been trying to get pregnant for a long time, the reality may make you scared; pregnancy in any case tends to make you over-emotional. You may also worry about the possibility of miscarriage and about whether your baby will be all right. All these fears are perfectly normal and should be discussed with your partner and, if you wish, with your doctor or midwife.

On a practical level you may wonder if you have the money, time or space for a child. If you include everything, up to and including college expenses, the cost of raising a child is staggering. But most people are able to handle it. It might be a good idea to start putting aside some money now, especially if you will be giving up work, and think about economies you can make in your living expenses.

For many women, the middle term of pregnancy is the most exhilarating time of their lives. Make the most of it: if you don't want to do certain things you have the perfect excuse for simply taking it easy. Alternatively, you may find you have enough energy for two during those weeks.

As you get more noticeably pregnant, friends will be full of advice. Listen to it all, but decide how much is relevant to you. Everyone is different and these forty weeks are a time for finding out about yourself.

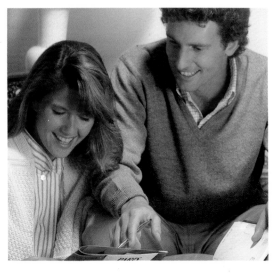

You may well become introspective during pregnancy. This is a good thing. Use the opportunity to rest, relax and get to know yourself. It will be the last time you have on your own for quite a while.

During pregnancy you may feel very romantic and should enjoy these feelings. Your partner no doubt will appreciate all the attention and affection and it may be some time after your baby is born before you feel so sensual again.

Towards the end of your pregnancy it is perfectly natural to feel impatient for it to be over, especially if you feel heavy, unattractive and uncomfortable. You may be filled with conflicting emotions: on the one hand anxious about having the child and giving birth, and yet on the other hand feeling that by now you can't wait to hold your baby. These emotions are perfectly understandable: a new member of your family is about to arrive and you are bound to feel a mixture of excitement together with a reasonable degree of nervousness.

This diary is intended to keep you company during your pregnancy. Use it to write your appointments in, scribble down your feelings, draw pictures of yourself and your belly, or write lists of babies' names. Most of all, try to enjoy your pregnancy. There's nothing left to say but "Good luck".

Week 2

Month: Dates:

MON

TUES

WED

THURS

FRI

SAT

SUN

Notes

Ovulation happens each month. It is when a ripe egg, or ovum – a single cell just 0.005in (0.13mm) large – is released from one of your ovaries and travels along your Fallopian tube. At the same time the lining of your womb becomes engorged with blood ready to receive and nourish an embryo and the mucus in your cervix becomes thinner so that sperm can swim through it more easily.

Most women ovulate about fourteen days before a period, whatever the length of their menstrual cycle. If you have an average twenty-eight day cycle, you will have ovulated on about the last day of this week – fourteen days from the first day of your last period.

An egg lives for about twenty-four hours after being released from the ovary, so if you are going to conceive, the egg has to be fertilized within these twenty-four hours. For you to be pregnant, you will have had sexual intercourse shortly before or after you ovulated and your ripe egg will have been fertilized by your partner's sperm. Except in the case of twins, only one sperm will pierce the outer coat of your egg and fertilize it. Instantly the egg loses its attraction, hardens its outer shell and all the other sperm drop off.

Most of the 400 million sperm ejaculated into your vagina (1) leak out, but some swim up through your cervix, into your uterus (2) and then into your Fallopian tube (3) The sperm are attracted to the ovum (4) and stick to its surface.

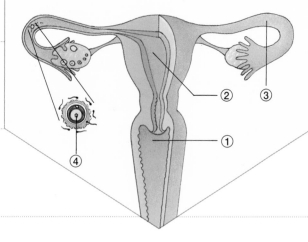

Pregnancy dangers

Once you know you are pregnant, it's time to become more aware of your body and learn to trust your intuition. You must consciously avoid all risks to your unborn child, which means coming to terms with the danger inherent in smoking, drinking and taking drugs. Their possible harmful effects are greatest during the first trimester of pregnancy, when the baby's organs are forming.

Smoking

It is extremely important that you stop smoking as soon as you know you are pregnant. Ask your partner to stop smoking too, to help you give up. Some women who smoke find that they develop a dislike of cigarettes early on in pregnancy; this may even be one of the first ways they know they are pregnant. If you find it impossible to stop smoking completely, at least cut right down.

Smoking during pregnancy increases the risk of early miscarriage and the chances of possible complications at birth – or of a stillborn baby. It has been proved that women who smoke ten or more cigarettes a day during pregnancy have smaller babies. Their children are also at greater risk of having a lower intellect or of being born with mental or physical abnormalities.

Alcohol

It is sensible to cut out alcohol completely, especially for the first three months of pregnancy. If you are planning to become pregnant, it is wise to cut down or stop drinking alcohol. Research shows that drinking alcohol, even in moderation, increases the risk of miscarriage or of a low-birthweight baby. It may also make physical abnormalities, heart defects or some degree of mental retardation more likely.

It obviously helps if you stop drinking alcohol during pregnancy, but even if you don't, cut out hard liquor completely, and restrict alcohol to an occasional glass of wine or beer.

Drugs

Don't take any drugs without consulting your doctor during pregnancy. Many drugs can cross the placenta and cause severe abnormalities in the fetus; even aspirin and sleeping tablets can be harmful, and very few antibiotics can be safely taken during the first three months of pregnancy. A few drugs do not cross the placenta and doctors are careful to prescribe only those known to be safe if you require treatment.

If you suffer from any illness or disorder for which you normally take drugs, tell your doctor if you are planning to become pregnant or immediately you suspect you may be pregnant – he or she may wish to change your course of treatment.

X-rays

Avoid X-rays if possible. If you do need to be X-rayed, it is important to stress that you are pregnant. A chest X-ray would be possible, for example, provided a lead apron was put over your stomach to prevent the rays reaching the baby.

German measles (rubella)

If you get German measles during the first three months of pregnancy your baby may be malformed, deaf, blind or born with heart disease. Rubella can also be the cause of miscarriage or stillbirth. Check whether you have been immunized against it, and keep well away from anyone who has German measles. Tell your doctor at once if you do come into contact with the disease.

How to stop smoking

- ☐ Think of your unborn baby, not just yourself.
- ☐ Tell everyone you are going to stop.
- ☐ Stop today – but keep a pack on you so you know you *could* start again.
- ☐ Put the money you would have spent on cigarettes in a glass jar so you can see how quickly it adds up.
- ☐ Change any habits related to cigarette smoking. Drink orange juice instead of tea or coffee (it's better for baby too).
- ☐ Avoid places where people are smoking.
- ☐ Keep your hands busy – start sewing or knitting baby clothes!
- ☐ If you become tense, breathe deeply and relax (see Week 29).
- ☐ Don't worry about not smoking forever, just worry about not smoking today.

Week 3

MON

TUES

WED

THURS

FRI

SAT

SUN

Notes

CONCEPTION

During the two weeks after fertilization, the cell that will become your baby multiplies quickly from a single-cell egg into over one hundred cells which will travel along your Fallopian tube until they reach your uterus.

Approximately thirty hours after fertilization, the fertilized cell divides into two identical cells. Roughly ten hours later these two cells divide again, making four cells in all. Within three days, the egg has divided into a total of sixteen cells, which get smaller and smaller with each division. At the same time, the cells are traveling along your Fallopian tube towards your uterus. By about the fourth day after fertilization, the egg, now a round, solid mass of over a hundred cells (and still growing), enters your uterus. It is now called a blastocyst and looks like a tiny blackberry. The blastocyst is formed of two layers: the outer one eventually becomes your placenta and the inner one, your embryo.

During the next few days the blastocyst floats free in the cavity of the uterus and is nurtured by "milk" secreted from the glands in the uterus lining. By the end of Week 3 the blastocyst will begin to attach itself firmly to your specially thickened womb lining, a process known as implantation. When this has happened, conception is said to have taken place.

Implantation usually takes place in the upper part of the uterus on either the left or right side, depending on which ovary ovulated.

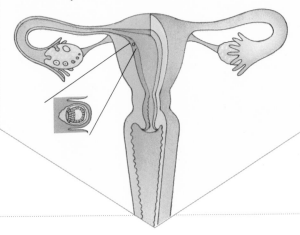

Healthy eating

During pregnancy remember that you are having to provide nutrition not only for yourself but also for your developing baby. This doesn't mean you should go overboard on quantity but that you should eat a good, varied, high-protein diet rich in vitamins and minerals – so start now. Eat fresh food whenever you can and try to cut out sweets, sodas, cakes, canned fruit, packaged desserts and soups, and chocolate.

Below is a suggested meal plan which you could easily follow during pregnancy. It contains 1,500 calories a day. (Your daily intake may well be more or less than this. Be guided by your own appetite and weight gain.) If you are hungry between meals eat raw vegetables or fresh fruit. If you follow a strict diet (vegetarian or macrobiotic), discuss this with your doctor: you may need to supplement it with extra minerals or vitamins (see Week 19). If you start feeling sick, follow the advice given in Week 7 and revert to this diet once the nausea is over.

What you need in your diet

Protein Pregnant women need at least 3oz of protein a day, especially if ill or tired. Eat two portions of meat or alternative (see Daily Allowances, right).

Carbohydrates These provide energy, but can make you fat. If you are overweight, eat wholewheat bread and avoid foods containing sugar, alcohol, white flour and rice.

Fiber Fiber (or roughage will help prevent constipation. Foods with high fiber content are peas and beans; wholewheat bread and cereals; potatoes (especially their skins); fruit, vegetables and nuts.

Fats Cut down on fats. Trim fat off meat; don't fry food or drown it in rich sauces; eat lowfat yogurt and milk.

Milk and dairy products Dairy products contain calcium which is important for your baby's development. The diet below will be sufficient for most women during pregnancy, but if you need building up you will need more dairy products.

Vitamins and minerals (see Week 19)

See Week 7 for advice on Morning Sickness

See Week 19 for Vitamins and Minerals

Daily allowances
Milk: ⅔ pint lowfat milk; lowfat cheese: 1oz; lowfat yogurt: 1oz; butter/margarine: ½oz; lowfat spread: 1oz.

Average portion of meat and alternatives
Meat: 3oz; white fish: 4oz; oily fish: 3oz; cottage cheese: 4oz; lowfat cheese: 3oz; 2 eggs; cooked lentils or beans: 6oz.

Average portion of bread and alternatives
Wholewheat bread (1 slice); 1 potato; 1 tablespoon cooked rice or pasta; 1 tablespoon yam, sweet potato, plantain; 1 carton plain yogurt; 1 extra serving fruit; 3 tablespoons wholegrain cereal; 2 wholewheat crackers.

Breakfast
Tomato juice or ½ fresh grapefruit
6 tablespoons wholegrain cereal or 2 slices wholewheat bread and butter from daily allowance (see above)
1 egg or small slice lean grilled bacon or fish
Milk from daily allowance
Mid-morning
Tea, coffee or low-calorie drink
1 fresh fruit or a small glass of fruit juice

Lunch
Clear soup or tomato juice
Average portion of meat or alternative
2 slices wholewheat bread or alternative (see above)
Large serving of vegetables or salad
1 fruit (as for mid-morning)
Afternoon
Tea, coffee or low-calorie drink
1 fruit (as for mid-morning)

Evening meal
Average portion of meat or alternative (see above)
2 slices wholewheat bread or alternative
Large serving of vegetables or salad
1 fruit (as for mid-morning)
1 low-fat yogurt or 1oz lowfat cheese
Bedtime
Tea, coffee or low-calorie drink

Week 4

Month: Dates:

MON

TUES

WED

THURS

FRI

SAT

SUN

Notes

You This is the week of your first missed period. You may be aware of some slight body changes.

Baby At the beginning of Week 4 your pregnancy is just a mass of cells embedded in the lining of your uterus, nourished by the blood vessels there. During Week 4 the cells multiply rapidly and group together to make different structures. The outer cells surrounding the embryo reach out like tree roots sending projections into the lining of your uterus. Those which penetrate deepest form the basis of the placenta.

At the same time the inner cells of the embryo form themselves into two, then three layers, each of which will grow to be different parts of your baby's body.

Other cells are developing into the amniotic sac. By the end of the week the embryo is completely embedded in the womb and is just visible to the naked eye.

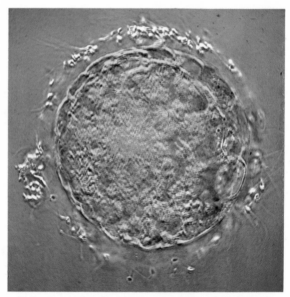

This mass of cells is an early stage of embryonic development. The surrounding pink ring is the debris of sperm that failed to penetrate the ovum.

Your due date

Medically your pregnancy is dated from the first day of your last period, and not from the time of conception. So, what is called "four weeks pregnant" is actually about two weeks after conception. Worked out like this, the average pregnancy lasts for forty weeks – the length of this diary. Use the chart below to work out the date your baby is due.

If your normal cycle is less than twenty-eight days, your due date or estimated date of confinement (EDC) will be a few days earlier than shown, since you ovulate earlier in a short menstrual cycle; conversely, in a cycle longer than twenty-eight days, you ovulate later and your due date will be a few days after the one shown in the chart.

Remember that this is just a rough guide – babies have a habit of arriving either early or late, hardly ever on time. Some people find it a good idea to give friends a due date about two weeks later than the actual one as it can be quite frustrating being constantly asked if the baby has arrived yet.

The trimesters

Pregnancy is divided into three trimesters (literally, thirds of pregnancy). The first is the first thirteen weeks, the second lasts from Week 14 to Week 27 and the third is from Week 28 until delivery.

The trimesters are a way of dividing up the forty weeks of pregnancy convenient to the medical profession, but you too will probably find that you naturally think of your pregnancy in three stages of roughly the same duration.

During the first trimester the fetus grows rapidly and all the different parts of the baby are formed. This is the period of greatest risk, both of miscarriage and of drugs causing congenital abnormalities. During the second and third trimesters the baby increases in size and his organs mature sufficiently for him to survive outside the womb. Many women feel at their best during the middle, or second trimester of their pregnancy.

See Week 7 for Morning Sickness

First signs

Morning sickness This is a misnomer. Many women feel sick all day or just in the evenings. Some women only *feel* sick, many actually are.

Tender breasts You may have already noticed your breasts becoming bigger and more sensitive as they can do before your period. They may also tingle slightly.

Exhaustion You may feel faint or dizzy or simply exhausted: try and rest.

Food and taste Some women experience a metallic taste in their mouth which affects their sense of taste. Others just stop eating some foods, commonly tea, coffee, alcohol, fatty and fried foods and fish. You may also get cravings for other foods.

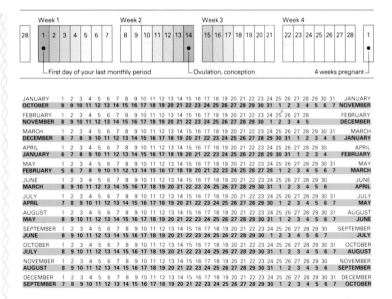

Menstrual calendar (top)
This shows a regular 28-day cycle. Your pregnancy is dated from the first day of your last period, although you conceived about two weeks later.

EDC chart (above)
To find your expected date of delivery, look at the first day of your last period on the top line of figures – your due date (EDC) appears in bold type beneath.

Week 5

Month: Dates:

MON

TUES

WED

THURS

FRI

SAT

SUN

Notes

You Week 5 is the first week that a urine test (which works by detecting a particular pregnancy hormone in your urine) would give you a positive result. The most likely sign of pregnancy is a missed period although you might mistake a little "breakthrough bleeding", which sometimes occurs, for an ordinary period. Other early signs of pregnancy that you may experience at some stage in the next few weeks are outlined in Week 4.

Baby Your baby's nervous system, spine and brain are already beginning to develop, and the cells which started off as an embryonic disc grow lengthways until your baby has a definite head and tail end.

The first stage in the development of the central nervous system is the formation of a groove in the top layer of cells towards the tail end of the embryo. The cells fold up and round to make the hollow neural tube, one end of which will become your baby's brain and the other end his spinal cord. At the same time blocks of tissue begin to grow which will eventually form your baby's spine, ribs and abdominal muscles.

During Week 5 your baby is shorter than your eyelashes – about 1/10in (2mm) – but he is rapidly developing his major component parts.

Star signs

Now you know approximately what date your baby is due, you might like to look at the star signs and see what characteristics he is likely to have – and what you might be letting yourself in for in terms of his possible future temperament!

The descriptions below are just little teasers. If you want an astrologer to tell you your baby's real character, and even possibly his future, you will need to know the exact time of his birth. Ask the nurse or your partner to keep an eye on the clock.

See Week 1 for kits for Pregnancy Tests

Capricorn
22 December–20 January
Serious, materialistic and ambitious, they rise through the ranks, but resist inner change. They are anxious for social prestige to bolster their ego, but always remain steadfast and reliable.

Taurus
21 April–21 May
Down-to-earth and sensual. They are sometimes slow starters, but always thorough. Taureans can be stubborn and possessive but are usually mild-tempered – except when they see red . . .

Virgo
24 August–22 September
Practical and hypercritical but well-intentioned; purist, perfectionist, perceptive – and tireless tidiers up. Always anxious to please, baby Virgo will bring you tea in bed in the morning.

Aquarius
21 January–18 February
Cerebral, intellectual, detached, they are the inventors and theoreticians of the ideal – although their ideals can be fairly fickle. They generate goodwill, friendship – and change.

Gemini
22 May–June 21
Versatile, verbal, mercurial – often concise and witty. They are usually as clever with their hands as with their tongues. Expect an intrepid traveler with an inquiring nature.

Libra
23 September–23 October
Attractive, tactful and poised. Innately artistic and such a sense of fairness, or indecision, that it is impossible for them not to take both sides of an argument.

Pisces
19 February–20 March
Innately psychic and finely attuned, both to the needs of living things and to music and poetry. They are liable to be injured, by their own need to be needed, and by dreamers of other dreams.

Cancer
22 June–22 July
Protective, nurturing, emotional; worriers; keepers of the past and of the familial dwelling. Not over-ambitious, your crab will give anything for a quiet, cozy life.

Scorpio
24 October–22 November
Secretive; jealous, demanding, revengeful and forever loyal once you are friendly; a real ability to get to the bottom of things . . . Scorpios are possibly a little paranoid.

Aries
21 March–20 April
Hot-tempered, passionate and aggressive; in battle, brave, indomitable and enthusiastic; likely to be either a trouble-maker or an initiator. Either way, he'll make sure he comes first.

Leo
23 July–23 August
Dramatic, charismatic, leonine. Warm-hearted and friendly, especially to those who appreciate them. You'll recognize your little Leo by his mane of hair and the way he purrs at himself in the mirror.

Sagittarius
23 November–21 December
Adventurous, both mentally and physically; expansive, sometimes over-indulgent, but philosophical and good-natured, with an open-door policy.

Week 6

Month: Dates:

MON

TUES

WED

THURS

FRI

SAT

SUN

Notes

You Whether or not you have done a pregnancy test at home, using a kit, you should at this stage visit your doctor to confirm your pregnancy. By now your uterus can be felt to be swollen and slightly enlarged – it is about the size of a tangerine.

Baby Although your baby's face still can't be made out, he already has a neck, a completed rudimentary brain and a bump for a head. The formation of the head is rapidly followed by the abdominal and chest cavities. In the chest cavity a heart is developing, which as yet has only two chambers instead of four.

This week the connecting stalk by which the embryo has been attached to your placenta begins to grow into the umbilical cord and blood vessels start forming within it, strengthening the link between you and your child. By the end of the week your baby has a bloodstream with a functioning circulation. Tiny limb buds appear at the corners of his body.

The lower part of the body is still comparatively undeveloped and looks more like a tail. Another shaping feature is that the blocks of tissue that make up the back of the embryo develop faster than those of the front, causing him to grow in a curved shape, resembling a seahorse.

By the end of this week your baby will be ¼in (6mm) long – the size of your little fingernail.

DON'T FORGET First doctor's visit to confirm your pregnancy.

Your relationship

If you have had a miscarriage or difficult pregnancies in the past or are experiencing vaginal bleeding now, ask your doctor's advice about sexual intercourse during the first fourteen weeks. The only other times not to have sex are at the very end of your pregnancy, either if you have a show (i.e. your plug of mucus is dislodged) or if your waters break. Otherwise there is no reason why you shouldn't have sexual intercourse throughout your pregnancy.

The only thing never to do in pregnancy is for your partner to blow into your vagina – this could lead to blood clots (embolism).

What if I feel frigid...?
The human female is one of the very few mammals to permit sexual intercourse at any time during pregnancy so it is not surprising if sometimes you don't feel like sex. If you do feel frigid during your pregnancy, don't worry – your desire will return later. A fairly typical pattern in pregnancy is for your sex drive to decrease in the first fourteen weeks then increase again in your second trimester (Weeks 14–27); you may lose interest in sex after about Week 29, as you get larger, more tired and uncomfortable.

See Week 1 for kits for Pregnancy Tests

See Week 4 for Your Due Date

See Week 9 for Prenatal Care

See Week 24 for Sex in Later Pregnancy

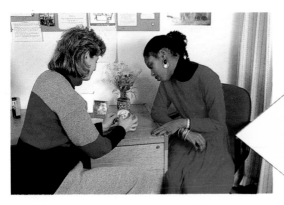

Seeing your doctor or midwife
You may not want to tell the world that you're pregnant just yet. But you must tell your doctor so that she can confirm your pregnancy and start you thinking about prenatal care.

Many women in fact feel highly sensual during pregnancy, especially during the second trimester. Your change in libido may be due to the high level of hormones circulating in your blood. During pregnancy your sexual organs are more highly developed and many parts of your body are more sensitive and therefore more capable of arousal. Sex could also be more fun now because it can be spontaneous – there's no worry about birth control or wondering whether this will lead to a longed-for baby.

Sexual superstitions
Contrary to what you or your partner may believe, it is impossible for his penis, or the semen which he ejaculates, to harm your baby. The muscles of the cervix and a special plug of mucus seal off your uterus completely. Where there is a risk (see above), the miscarriage could be triggered off by your orgasm causing your uterus to contract, which might set off other contractions. But this will not happen in a normal pregnancy.

First visit to doctor or midwife
Your first prenatal visit should include a complete physical examination and the taking of a full medical history. Your caregiver will review your general health and ask you if you have ever had illnesses that could affect your baby's health, such as high blood pressure, heart disease or diabetes. You will also be asked for the first date of your last menstrual period, so that your baby's due date can be determined. An ultrasound examination may be done to corroborate the baby's gestational age (see Ultrasound scan, p. 37). Blood and urine samples will be taken to determine blood type and run routine laboratory tests for Rh factor, anemia, syphilis, immunity to German measles, and gestational diabetes, among other things.

Be sure to ask about obstetrical fees and hospital costs and find out what your insurance covers.

17

Week 7

Month: _____ Dates: _____

MON

TUES

WED

THURS

FRI

SAT

SUN

Notes

▮ YOU AND YOUR DEVELOPING BABY

You You may feel dizzy or faint if you stand for long periods. You may also have spells of overwhelming tiredness, which is normal. Go to bed earlier at night and, if possible, rest during the day. By now you may be experiencing some of pregnancy's 'problems', including some emotional ones.

Baby Week 7 is when many begin to call the embryo a fetus. Although your baby's head still has some strange-looking lumps and is still at an unusual angle to its body, being bent forward on its chest, it is beginning to assume its eventual human shape. The limb buds are growing rapidly and arms and legs starting to resemble paddle-shapes.

The ears and eyes are developing and apertures for the nostrils are appearing. Development of the jaws and mouth is continuing and the lips, tongue and first teeth buds are now visible.

By the end of this week your baby's brain and spinal cord will be almost complete. The heart, although still a simple structure, now has four chambers. It is beating with enough force to circulate blood cells through the complex network of blood vessels that extends into the head and throughout the body.

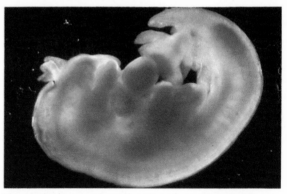

Your baby is now about the size of your thumbnail.

▮ **DON'T FORGET** Start investigating prenatal classes (See Week 29) if you haven't already.

Mixed emotions

You will be coming to terms with what it means to be pregnant. From initial excitement or nervousness, your feelings may be settling into a state of contentment. It is up to you when you announce to the world that you are pregnant. Some want to broadcast the news as soon as the pregnancy is confirmed, while others prefer to wait until they are sure all is well, after three months or so.

The first trimester may well be the worst time of your pregnancy, emotionally as well as physically. You have just taken a step into the unknown which is, let's face it, quite courageous. No matter how much you may have wanted a baby in the past, you may now be wondering if you've made the right decision. Possibly for the first time in your life, you are also being forced into a constant awareness of your body which may be making you feel sick, tired and over-emotional. You may also be a bit nervous that you are going to miscarry.

It can seem that you are surrounded by pregnant women, and you may find everyone will want to tell you their pregnancy stories. Listen if you want to and don't if you prefer not. Always trust your own instincts.

Allaying your fears

It's quite normal to worry about whether your baby is going to be all right and whether anything you're doing might harm him. Thankfully only a tiny percentage of babies born today are handicapped. It is important to behave sensibly throughout your pregnancy; keep all your doctor's appointments and never be afraid to ask for medical advice on anything that is worrying you (see Week 9): remember that you're asking for your baby as well as for yourself. Cut down on any risks to your baby such as smoking or drinking (see Week 2).

Most women are worried about labor. Dreams about giving birth to weird objects are common. You may find it helps sharing your fears about labor with your friends or your doctor or midwife. On a broader level, you may feel worried about how the baby is going to change your life, both financially and socially. Will it end your freedom? Disrupt the happy relationship you have with your partner? You may wonder how you will cope with bringing up a child. Note down your anxieties and feelings in this diary – you'll be amazed how the worries increase and decrease in importance during the weeks ahead. Never let a problem get you down – find someone to discuss it with.

At times during your pregnancy you may have the sense of being very alone and feel that your partner isn't doing enough. You may argue more during pregnancy, but you will also feel closer. Much of this can be put down to changing hormones. It is important to involve your partner as early as you can.

See Weeks 11 and 12 for Common Problems

See Week 23 for The Father's Role

Morning sickness

By now you may have begun to feel sick. Nausea, and sometimes actual vomiting, affects about half of all pregnant women and you may feel sick at any time, day or night. The cause is thought to be related to the hormonal changes taking place in your body. Morning sickness is not serious, just very unpleasant, but with luck it will disappear around the twelfth to fourteenth week – let your doctor know if you are still nauseous after Week 14.

If you can't keep anything down, not even drinks, tell your doctor. But otherwise, try to alleviate the symptoms and reduce the risk of being sick. Here are some suggestions that may help.

☐ Eat a cracker before getting out of bed in the morning and get up slowly.

☐ Have a bowl of cereal and milk before you go to sleep.

☐ Eat small, light meals – as many as you need – throughout the day. Try half a baked potato or sipping soda water as stomach settlers.

☐ Drink fluids between meals rather than with food.

☐ Wear clothes without waistbands.

☐ Put away anything that makes you feel sick, such as soaps or perfume.

☐ If cooking smells make you nauseous, buy foods that don't need preparing.

DIC 12 '8 weeks 95/m

Week 8

Month: _____ Dates: _____

MON

TUES

WED

THURS

FRI

SAT 8 weeks
Nov. 28 2002

SUN

Notes

You You may already start to notice your body changing. Your waist may be vanishing, and your breasts and nipples will be enlarging.

Baby Week 8 is an important time for the growth of your baby's eyes and inner ear. At the moment the eyes are covered by a skin which will eventually split to form eyelids. His ears are visible but not yet protruding. The middle part of the ear, responsible for balance as well as hearing, will have developed by the end of the week. During the next seven days he will start to open his mouth and be able to suck and chew once the upper and lower jaws fuse at the sides.

By now his heart is pumping vigorously with a regular rhythm. Blood vessels can be seen through the skin which is as thin as tracing paper. All the major internal organs (heart, brain, lungs, kidneys, liver and intestine) are now in place although not yet fully developed.

The bones of his arms and legs are starting to harden and elongate; fingers and toes are more obvious though joined by webs of skin; and the major joints (shoulders, elbows, hips and knees) are forming.

At present your baby is still smaller than your nose – 1in (2.5cm) long – and fish-like in shape, with an over-large head and small body.

■ **DON'T FORGET** Make a dental appointment. Buy a support bra soon.

Looking good

A good diet, plus plenty of rest and sleep, are extremely important throughout pregnancy. Experiment with make-up and different hairstyles if you want people to look at your face rather than your stomach. You may well find you look better than ever over the next few months.

Hair Both hair and nails grow more rapidly than usual. Dry hair may become drier and greasy hair greasier. Don't experiment with perms or color just now. Short hair is more manageable and easier to wash.

Nails Nails may break or split easily. Keep them short and wear gloves for any chores. Try rubbing baby oil into the base of your nails nightly to help prevent cracking, and eat more dairy products.

Breasts Don't use soap on your breasts. To toughen your nipples before breast-feeding, try splashing your breasts every morning with lots of cold water or rubbing your nipples daily with a washcloth. Buy two new support bras (see below).

Skin Most women's skin improves but if yours does the opposite, don't worry – after pregnancy it will be back to normal. The extra blood circulating round your body will make you look rosy-cheeked and 'blooming'. Use moisturizer but not foundation creams; let the new color of your skin shine through.

Stretch marks These may occur if the elastic fibers in your skin have become over-stretched and ruptured. Although they first appear as dramatic reddish streaks, they shrink to indistinct silvery lines afterwards. There is no sure way to avoid stretch marks. It helps not to put on too much weight and to maintain a correct posture. Applying special body creams will also help to keep your skin supple. You can get support for your abdomen from a lightweight pregnancy corset.

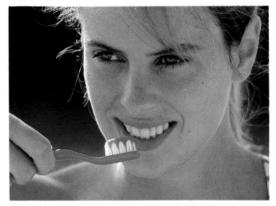

Color changes Pigmented birthmarks and freckles can darken during pregnancy, especially if exposed to sunlight. They will lighten again after delivery. Some women may get blotchy patches on their face and neck; these are caused by pregnancy hormones. Use make-up to cover them up if they worry you. They will start to disappear after delivery.

Teeth During pregnancy the gums around your teeth become spongier and more prone to infection – you may notice them bleeding more. Avoid sugary foods, brush your teeth at least twice a day and floss them regularly. Make an appointment with your dentist now and don't forget to tell him or her that you are pregnant.

Personal hygiene You may find you sweat more, due to an increase in body weight and temperature. Wash regularly and wear cotton underwear if possible; use talcum powder after washing. Never douche during pregnancy.

Buying a new bra
Your breasts may increase by as much as two bra sizes during pregnancy. Since breasts contain no muscular tissue, they need good support or they may never return to their normal shape.

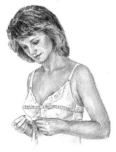

It is a good idea to go to a shop where staff are trained to fit bras. They should have wide shoulder straps and adjustable backs to allow for later chest expansion. Make sure they are the right cup size.

Week 9

Month: Dates:

MON

TUES

WED

THURS

FRI

SAT

SUN

Notes

You You may begin to notice skin changes caused by pregnancy hormones. Any wrinkles may become less obvious due to your face fattening out. Your gums may also be thickening. Gingivitis or gum infection is more common during pregnancy (see Week 8). Start some regular exercise; go walking or swimming every day if possible, though avoid swimming around the time you would normally be expecting your period. Diving is not recommended during pregnancy.

Baby Your baby is beginning to have a more mature appearance although his head is still bent forward on his chest. The development of his eyes is now complete, although each eye still has a membrane eyelid over it. A nose has also appeared.

During Week 9 the chest cavity becomes separated from the abdominal cavity by a band of muscle that later develops into the diaphragm, a muscle that plays an important role in breathing. The spine is making its first, tiny movements and, although you won't be able to feel it yet, your baby is starting to kick and move around in order to exercise his muscles.

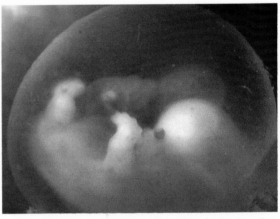

The fastest growth this week is in the limbs, hands and feet. Fingers and toes start to be defined.

Prenatal care

Regular prenatal checkups should start by Week 12 of your pregnancy. They should take place monthly, and more frequently in the last two months before delivery. These checkups are essential to give your baby the best start in life; studies have shown that regular prenatal care helps prevent complications of pregnancy and birth. They also give you an opportunity to ask questions and air your concerns. So no matter what you may feel, or how busy you are – for your sake and your baby's – keep your appointments!

Write down everything you want to discuss with your doctor or midwife before every visit – it is easy to forget things once you are there (pregnancy amnesia is famous!). If they are short of time, ask when you can come back for a discussion. It is important that you find answers to everything that is worrying you. Take notes of the discussion or you may forget what the doctor said.

Think about the kind of birth you want before you start talking to your doctor or midwife about it. Read books about childbirth and talk to friends about the birth of their children. It is most important that you are happy when giving birth.

Below is a list of questions you may wish to ask. They apply mainly to hospital deliveries.

See Week 35 for Pain Relief

See Week 40 for The Birth

See page 88 for Understanding your Medical Records

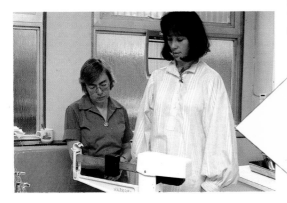

Prenatal checkups
You will be weighed at each visit, to check that your baby is growing satisfactorily and that you are not putting on too much weight. Your blood pressure will be measured each time and a sample of urine tested.

Questions for the doctor and hospital

Prenatal care
- ☐ How often will I have prenatal appointments?
- ☐ What tests will you be giving me?
- ☐ Where can I go for prenatal classes?
- ☐ Will I be shown around the labor and maternity wards before the birth?

The birth
- ☐ Is my partner (or close relative or friend) welcome all the time during labor?
- ☐ Will they ever be asked to leave the room? If so, why?
- ☐ What is your policy on induction, pain relief, episiotomy, routine monitoring?
- ☐ Is an epidural available?
- ☐ Do you automatically shave my pubic hair or give me an enema?
- ☐ Can I walk around in labor and find my own position for birth?
- ☐ If I need to have a Cesarean section can my partner stay with me? Can it be done with an epidural?
- ☐ Will my baby be put to my breast immediately after birth?
- ☐ Is it possible to be alone with my baby and partner immediately after the birth?

The hospital
- ☐ Do you have a Special Care Unit? If not, where is the nearest one?
- ☐ Do you have a birthing chair, a birthing pool (or any other equipment you want to know about)?
- ☐ Is it possible to have my baby born in subdued lighting and a quiet atmosphere?
- ☐ What is the normal length of stay on the maternity ward?
- ☐ How many beds are there to a room?
- ☐ What are visiting hours?
- ☐ Are there any special rules about visiting or about numbers of visitors?

Week 10

MON

TUES

WED

THURS

FRI

SAT

SUN

Notes

YOU AND YOUR DEVELOPING BABY

You Your uterus has now grown to the size of an orange but is still hidden away within your pelvis. Your heart, lungs and kidneys are also beginning to work harder; start watching your diet (see Week 3) particularly carefully. Your breasts will be noticeably larger by now and can be rather tender.

Baby During the last four weeks your baby's brain has developed so rapidly that his head is still large in proportion to the rest of his body. By the end of this week the inner part of the ears are complete and the external parts are beginning to grow.

The lungs are growing inside the chest cavity and, in the abdomen, the stomach and intestine are formed and the kidneys are moving into their permanent positions. The umbilical cord is properly formed and blood is circulating along it.

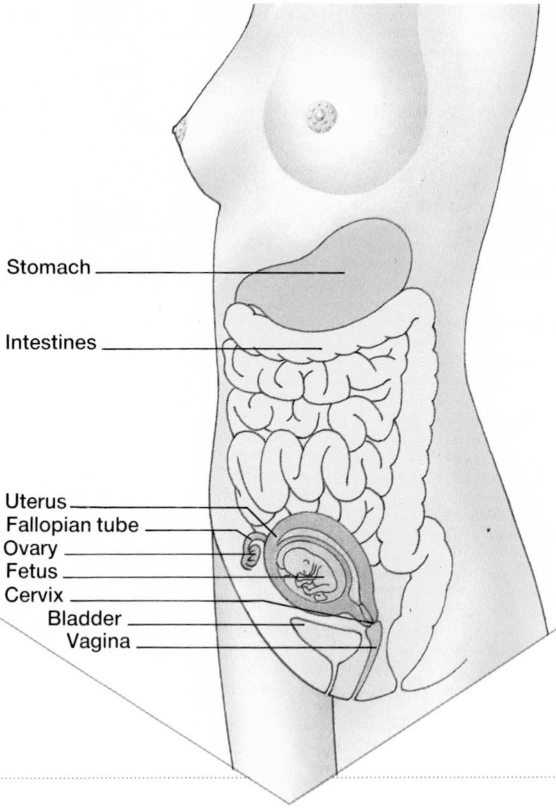

Stomach

Intestines

Uterus
Fallopian tube
Ovary
Fetus
Cervix
Bladder
Vagina

DON'T FORGET Find out now about your employer's maternity leave policy if you haven't already.

Working in pregnancy

One positive advantage of working during pregnancy is that it takes your mind off waiting. But if your job is potentially dangerous (involving a lot of bending or heavy lifting, contact with chemicals, lead, dangerous substances or X-rays), it is best to discuss with your doctor and employer about how safe it is to continue. If it normally involves a lot of standing, see if you can switch to a more sedentary job for the time being. If there is *any* medical reason why you should stop work, then do, but remember that you will need a doctor's certificate. If you have any problems with your employer, try and get legal help (see below).

See Week 7 for Morning Sickness

Sleepiness may make it impossible for you to concentrate during early pregnancy. For many this is the most difficult time in which to work. Don't push yourself – this feeling of exhaustion will only last for another few weeks. If you find yourself dropping off to sleep during the day, you need rest. Try and take some time off work until you feel less tired. Nausea may also make it hard to concentrate. Bring in food to pick at during the day to stop you feeling sick and make sure you have a good breakfast.

If you have a medical complication during pregnancy and need to take more time off than your employers allows, you will need your physician's help in applying for disability benefits. Talk with your doctor and the personnel officer where you work for guidance about this.

Working after childbirth

Around this time you should start thinking about whether you do want to return to work (either full- or part-time) after you have had your baby and, if you do, how long you want to take on maternity leave. Discuss all this with your partner and, subsequently, your employer. It is wise to confirm your arrangements in writing.

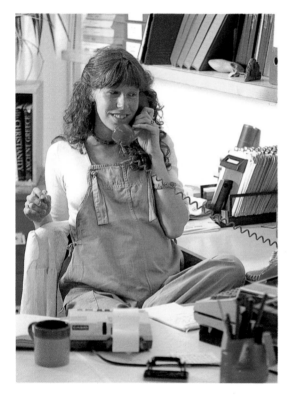

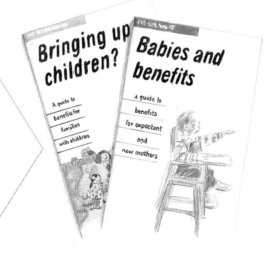

The Pregnancy Discrimination Act

The Pregnancy Discrimination Act (an amendment to Title VII of the 1964 Civil Rights Act) prohibits discrimination against employees on the basis of pregnancy, childbirth and related medical conditions. But the law does not require an employer to provide a specific number of weeks for maternity leave or establish new benefit programs where none exist. Check the employee handbook before discussing your situation with the personnel officer.

Week 11

Month: Dates:

MON

TUES

WED

THURS

FRI

SAT

SUN

Notes

You If you've been feeling sick during the last few weeks you may begin to feel better. Start thinking about where you want to go for prenatal classes and book now as they often fill up early (see Week 29).

Baby By the end of the week all your baby's essential internal organs will be formed and the majority beginning to function. From now on, these organs will simply continue to grow in size. From the end of Week 11, therefore, your baby is relatively safe from the risk of developing major congenital abnormalities.

His head is still relatively large for his body size and his limbs are still quite short and thin. His ankles and wrists have formed and his elbows and knees are taking shape.

By the end of this week, however, he is clearly recognizable as a small human baby. His face is also beginning to look more human as it becomes more rounded. The back of the head has enlarged, so that his eyes are in a more natural position; his ears look flatter and continue to develop.

Your baby's heart is pumping blood to all parts of the body as well as through the umbilical cord to what will eventually become the placenta.

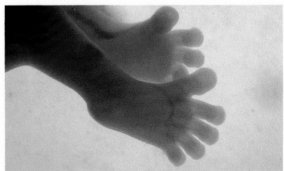

Your baby's fingers and toes are now separate and clearly developed.

■ **DON'T FORGET** Go and see your dentist if you haven't already.

Common problems/1

Most of the problems mentioned here and in Week 12 are fairly common in early pregnancy and are more of a nuisance than serious. Speak to your doctor immediately, however, if you experience any of the problems highlighted in the panel.

Backache See Week 31
Bladder problems In early and late pregnancy you need to urinate more frequently, sometimes to the extent that it wakes you up at night. You could try drinking less in the evening and rocking back and forwards as you urinate, which lessens the pressure on your bladder and may help empty it more completely. Talk to your doctor if you have pain or blood when urinating. (See also Cystitis below)
Bleeding gums This can be a sign of gum infection (gingivitis). Pregnancy is an important time for dental hygiene (see Week 8). Massage your gums with fingertips before brushing your teeth, using a soft bristle brush. See your dentist.
Blocked nose Your nose may be more stuffed-up than usual, especially on waking up. Don't blow your nose too hard and don't use a nasal spray or take cold cures for it. Avoid dusty atmospheres and try menthol or plain steam inhalations. Your blocked nose will probably disappear after childbirth if not before. (See also Nose bleeds, Week 12)
Constipation This may last throughout your pregnancy, due to the hormone progesterone causing your intestinal muscles to relax,

Contact the doctor if you:
- ☐ Are vomiting excessively.
- ☐ Have abdominal cramps.
- ☐ Have any vaginal bleeding apart from around the time of your first missed period.
- ☐ Have any leak of clear fluid from your vagina.
- ☐ Fall or have an accident.
- ☐ Have swollen feet, fingers, ankles or face.
- ☐ Are short of breath.
- ☐ Have excessive dizziness or headaches.
- ☐ Don't notice any fetal movements for twenty-four hours or more.
- ☐ Have excessive white or discolored discharge

which slows down your bowel movements. Drink lots of water and fruit juice and eat bran and wholewheat bread. Avoid strong laxatives and go to the bathroom the moment you feel you need to: too much straining could lead to piles (see Week 12).
Cramps Cramps may be due to poor blood circulation, lack of salt in the diet or having hot milky drinks before bed. It usually occurs in your legs. If it happens at night, try hopping on the foot of the affected leg or massaging it firmly for a while – or stretch the affected part, then quickly bend it. Make sure your bedding is loose.

If you get a lot of cramps, try going for a short walk or try and stretch your calf muscles by exercising your legs in some other way before you go to bed to get the circulation going. Your doctor may give you calcium supplements.

Cystitis (bladder infection) If you have a burning feeling when urinating and you feel as if you have to urinate all the time, you may have cystitis. See your doctor immediately and drink as much water as you can.
Fainting During early and late pregnancy you may feel dizzy or unsteady and may even faint, due to the brain being relatively deprived of blood, because your blood is rushing either to your feet (if you are standing) or to your uterus. If you feel faint get into fresh air as soon as possible, loosen tight clothes and sit down or, if possible, lie down with your head flat and your legs raised. Don't lock the bathroom door if you are at home.

Avoid standing for long periods, having hot baths, sitting in smoky atmospheres and getting up too quickly from a sitting or lying position. Try increasing your iron intake (see Week 19).
Flatulence This is due to a sluggish intestine during pregnancy. Flatulence is caused either by you swallowing air (often to stop yourself feeling sick) or eating certain foods (like beans, fried foods, cabbage, onions and peppers). Avoid problem foods where possible and eat light meals.
Headaches Try not to worry if you get occasional headaches; rest and relaxation help. If your headaches are frequent, tell your doctor – it may be a sign of high blood pressure.
Hemorrhoids See Piles
Incontinence See Week 24
Indigestion and heartburn See Week 24

See Week 24 for Problems of Later Pregnancy

(Continued in Week 12)

27

Week 12

Month: Dates:

MON

TUES

WED

THURS

FRI

SAT

SUN

Notes

You Your uterus can now be felt as a hard ridge above your pubic bone, although you may not yet know what you are feeling for. From the beginning of this week you will probably start putting on serious weight. About a quarter of your pregnancy weight gain will take place from now until Week 20 (see Week 25). Most women gain 15–30lb. If you are underweight now, you may need to put on more than 30lb. If you are overweight, it may be a good idea to discuss a diet with your doctor to make sure you put on less than 30lb (see Week 3). Never start an unsupervised diet while pregnant.

Baby Although few muscles are working, your baby is already using the muscles that will be used in breathing after birth. His brain and muscles are coordinating so that he is kicking, curling his toes, rotating his feet and wrists, clenching and unclenching his fists, pressing his lips together, frowning and making other facial expressions.

This week the umbilical cord starts to circulate blood between the fetus and the group of membranes attached to the wall of your uterus. Your baby begins to rely on these membranes for nourishment and the placenta (or afterbirth) now begins to function.

Common problems/2

Insomnia Don't worry about not sleeping; it's more important that you relax. Try the usual tricks – a warm milk drink at bedtime (unless you are suffering from cramps); reading a good book; having a warm bath; relaxation exercises (see Week 33). If insomnia becomes a problem, talk to your doctor about it – don't take sleeping pills without advice.

Itching and skin problems General itching – with or without a rash – can be due to poor hygiene, excess weight gain and/or sweating. Keep your body clean and apply calamine lotion or talcum powder to the affected area. Try and keep cool – wear loose clothing (no waistbands) made of natural fibers. Any tiny red spots, or naevi, in your skin are harmless and will disappear.

Morning sickness See Week 7

Nose bleeds During pregnancy there is an increased volume of blood in your body, including in the vessels lining your nose. Nose bleeds can easily occur if you blow your nose too hard and the vessels rupture. If you are subject to nose-bleeding, try breathing through your mouth and avoid blowing your nose violently. If your nose starts bleeding, lean forward slightly and apply gentle pressure to the bridge of your nose, or pinch your nostrils together to stop the blood flow.

Piles (hemorrhoids) Piles are a form of varicose vein which occur around the anus. You may first notice some discomfort and possibly some bleeding when you have a bowel movement. Piles can be caused by anything that increases pressure in your abdomen such as constipation, chronic coughing or lifting. They can be very uncomfortable, especially when passing stools, and they may itch and bleed slightly especially if the pile is large and outside your rectum. Cure your constipation (see Week 11) and try to keep your stools soft and regular. Keep your anal area clean to avoid irritation and ask your doctor for creams or suppositories if you need help.

If your piles itch badly, put some crushed ice in a plastic bag, cover it with a cloth and hold the pack gently against the piles. Piles usually go within a week or two of delivery.

Pins and needles See Week 24

Stretch marks See Week 8

Sweating Wash frequently and use talcum powder. Wear natural fibers and drink more to replace lost fluids.

Swelling of legs, ankles, fingers (Edema) See Week 24

Thrush Thrush is common during pregnancy and can be passed on to your baby, although this can be quickly cleared up by a course of medicine. Don't wear panty hose or panties that are too tight; ask your doctor for creams and suppositories to clear up the infection.

Tiredness This may go on throughout pregnancy although it often gets better in your second trimester.

Vaginal secretions An increase in vaginal secretions is normal during pregnancy due to the change in vaginal tissues in preparation for the birth. If your secretions smell awful, make you sore, are painful or contain blood, tell your doctor. Otherwise, if you need to, wear a sanitary napkin (not a tampon) and in any case wear cotton underwear and wash often. Never douche or use a vaginal deodorant during pregnancy. Make sure you don't have thrush (see above).

Varicose veins Varicose veins can be inherited or caused by hormones or, in later pregnancy, by your enlarged womb pressing down and obstructing the flow of blood from your legs to your heart.

Avoid standing or sitting still for long periods, crossing your legs, wearing tight garments or being constipated. If varicose veins do run in the family, wear support hose or stockings from an early age.

To prevent varicose veins, exercise frequently, watch your weight and rest every day with legs raised above your heart.

See Week 24 for Problems of Later Pregnancy

It is most important to rest when you feel tired in pregnancy.

Week 13

Month: Dates:

MON

TUES

WED

THURS

FRI

SAT

SUN

Notes

You From now on your uterus will be enlarging at a noticeable rate. It is already swollen by your pregnancy and measures approximately 4in in diameter. Your doctor will be able to feel it in your lower abdomen as a soft swelling coming out of your pelvis.

The main danger of miscarriage is over. From now on syphilis, rubella (German measles) and rare tropical diseases are the only known infections which can cross to the fetus and do him any harm.

You may see a dark line (the *linea nigra*) appearing down the center of your abdomen. This continues to darken during pregnancy but will fade after delivery.

Baby By the end of this week your baby is properly formed. But were he to be born, he could not survive because, although all the organs are present, they have not yet matured enough to perform the jobs for which they are intended. The rest of your pregnancy is designed to allow the fetus to grow in size, and to give his vital organs sufficient time to mature so that they are capable of independent life.

His neck is now fully developed, which allows his head to move freely on his body. His face is formed, with mouth, nose and external ears properly developed.

By the end of this week your baby is 3in long and weighs 1oz. He has plenty of room to move within the amniotic sac.

The hereditary factor

It is only natural to fantasize about what your child will be like. Your genes – the basic elements that control heredity – in combination with your partner's will determine a great deal about your child, although environment will also play a large part. There are 23 pairs of chromosomes in every cell in the human body except for the sperm cell and the egg cell, each of which contains only 23. Each chromosome consists of tiny segments called genes, and each gene is responsible for a specific characteristic such as hair color or the shape of the eye.

At conception, the specific genes of the father line up with similar genes of the mother. Which characteristic the child inherits depends on which of the two genes is stronger, or dominant, and which is weaker, or recessive. For example, a brown hair gene is dominant over a light blond hair gene. If these two genes meet, the child will have brown hair. However, if two light blond hair genes meet, the child will have light blond hair. Since each person carries in his cells the genes of his close relatives as well as his parents, a child may inherit qualities not apparent in either of his parents. So two dark-haired parents could still, for instance, have a blond-haired child.

Genetic counseling and testing is now available for parents who are concerned about passing on to their children some disease which has occurred in their family background. Ask your doctor for more information, or, to locate the genetic counseling and testing center nearest you, contact the National Center for Education in Maternal and Child Health (see Useful Addresses p.92).

Choosing a name for your baby
All parents want to choose the "perfect" name for their child. And for many people, this quest can become one of the most amusing and sometimes agonizing pastimes of all during pregnancy.

Your choice of a name will probably be influenced greatly by family tradition and sentimental associations. But how the name sounds and looks are also important considerations. The longer and more arresting the family name, the shorter and simpler the first name should be. As a rule, one or two-syllable first names fit best with three-syllable last names; for example, Ann Markowitz is better than Anita Markowitz and a one-syllable family name calls for a polysyllabic first name, such as Eugenia Smith or Alexander Jones.

Herbs during pregnancy
If you don't feel like drinking coffee or caffeine-containing teas and soft drinks, you may want to try herb teas. Most herbs and herbal teas (especially prepackaged ones) cannot harm you if taken in moderation, but some can contain chemically active substances which may be harmful. For example, the herbs such as pennyroyal, mugwort, tansy, cohosh, slippery elm can have an unwanted action on the uterus. Some herbs, such as sage, marjoram and parsley, are safe during pregnancy in the amounts used in cooking but should not be taken in larger quantities. It's best to be certain of the properties of any herbs you use. Consult a book on herbal pharmacology at the library if you are not sure.

Week 14

Month: Dates:

MON

TUES

WED

THURS

FRI

SAT

SUN

Notes

You You are beginning the middle stage of your pregnancy, generally thought of as the most enjoyable. During the next fourteen weeks you will probably feel better, more creative and more energetic, as well as more positive about your new baby, than at any other stage of pregnancy. Your uterus is now the size of a large grapefruit and you should be able to feel the top of it two fingers' breadth above your pubic bone.

Baby Week 14 is the beginning of the second trimester, the stage of the main growth of your baby; he increases in size, his organs mature and complex hormone and other processes develop.

Your baby has begun to grow hair: he has eyebrows and a small amount of hair on his head. His heart is beating strongly and can be heard using an ultrasonic device. His heartbeat is almost twice the rate of a normal adult's. All his major muscles are responding to stimulation from the brain. The arms can bend from the wrist and elbow, the fingers can curl, make fists and grasp: his nervous system has begun to function.

Your placenta is now fully operational; it both nourishes your fetus and produces hormones. Your child starts to drink some amniotic fluid and his kidneys begin to make a little urine which he can now pass.

During the last seven days your baby has more than doubled in weight. He now weighs 2$\frac{1}{4}$oz and measures about 4in.

Other children

Looking after children is one of the most exhausting occupations for a pregnant woman. Learn to pick up your child with your knees bent, or kneel down to cuddle and comfort him instead of picking him up. Make an effort to stay cool, calm and collected, especially during early pregnancy, and try not to let your attitude to your older children change.

If possible, don't talk about your pregnancy to your children too soon or they will get bored with waiting. Only once they have noticed, should they be told that a baby is growing inside your stomach. Later on, go through this diary with them week by week, and let them feel him kicking inside you.

Prepare children by pointing out babies in their carriages in the street – comment on how helpless they look so that the new baby is not expected to be a playmate from the start. Show older children pictures of themselves as babies and buy them dolls of their own so they have someone to look after too. Shortly before the event, take them to buy their new sibling a present. If you need a

The middle term of pregnancy

Emotions The middle period of pregnancy is usually a time for feeling positive, energetic and creative. You may begin to feel closer to other women and find yourself talking about personal things you haven't discussed before. You may love the attention you receive from other people once they notice your pregnancy.

The first time your baby kicks can be very exciting and may bring you much closer to him. It's the first real sign that someone separate from you is there, and that something really is happening.

Working Your excess energy can make you overdo things during your working day. No matter how strong you feel, take it easy whenever you can. Skip lunch dates and lunchtime shopping expeditions: instead bring in a salad and sandwich for lunch. Don't stand all day – this may lead to circulation problems and varicose veins later on. Put your feet up when you can – rest them on the drawer of your filing cabinet or on your wastepaper basket. Try squatting instead of bending over which might strain your back. Always ask for help – people are happy to give it.

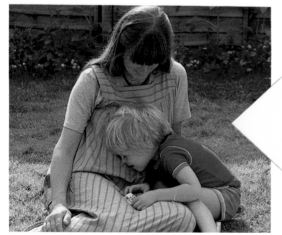

Involving older children
Children should be encouraged to want a brother or sister and, later, to care for the new baby so that they feel involved rather than resentful. Inform and involve them in your pregnancy too, according to their age and how much they can understand.

child to move out of his familiar crib, or room, do it well before the baby is born so that the two events do not appear related. Let your partner increase his involvement with your children, especially with bathing, feeding and story-telling, so that you can decrease yours well before the birth.

If you are having the baby in the hospital, make arrangements for your children well in advance and rehearse their timetables and movements frequently; it is only surprise that will worry them. When you leave for the hospital, say goodbye to them no matter what time it is. It is upsetting for children to wake up and find you gone.

If you want a home birth, your children will be involved right from the start. Tell them what is going to happen beforehand.

Week 15

Month: _____ Dates: _____

MON

TUES

WED

THURS

FRI

SAT

SUN

Notes

You Your clothes are probably getting too tight for you and you will need to wear looser garments. Your pregnancy may even begin to show, though this varies a lot from person to person. To cope with the increased amount of blood circulating in your body and your baby's need for oxygen, your enlarged heart has increased its output by twenty per cent. You're probably beginning to feel more energetic, so think about a vacation sometime during the next ten weeks.

Baby From now on most of your baby's energy is directed towards growing and maturing. The hair on his head is becoming thicker and he now has eyelashes as well as eyebrows. The three tiny bones of his middle ear are the first bones to harden, which means he is probably capable of hearing, although the auditory centers in his brain, which make sense of sounds received, have not yet developed. The amniotic fluid that surrounds him is an excellent sound conductor and from now on he will hear your stomach rumbling, your heart beating and the sound of your voice, as well as occasional noises from outside the womb.

The baby now measures approximately 5¼in and weighs roughly 3½oz.

■ **DON'T FORGET** Start exercising regularly if you haven't already. Add abdominal and pelvic floor exercises to your regimen.

Vacations

You may find that your nesting instinct is very strong during pregnancy and you are happiest staying in your home environment. But if it is your first child you're probably only too aware that this may be your last opportunity for a vacation alone together for a while. But where? And when?

Avoid doing too much traveling during pregnancy as it can be tiring even if you are not driving. Try to plan an enjoyable but essentially restful vacation: relax by a swimming pool or escape to the heart of the countryside. Enjoy the company of your partner.

When is the best time to go away?
First trimester Nausea, vomiting and tiredness may stop you enjoying any travel. If you have to travel, do so in that part of the day when you feel best.
Second trimester This is the best time to go away during pregnancy – especially between Weeks 20 and 27 – although you may still get uncomfortable and restless if you have to sit in cramped conditions on a journey. Walk around as much as you can to keep your circulation going. Your feet are likely to swell on plane journeys, so wear shoes that give.

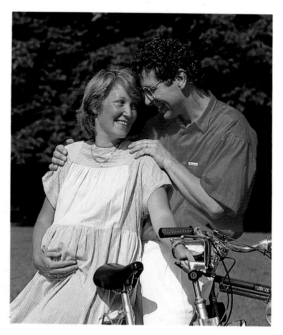

See
Week 17 for
Pelvic Floor
Exercises

See
Weeks 21
and 22 for
Keeping Fit

Third trimester It is advisable not to go on any long trips towards the end of pregnancy. Car journeys lasting an hour or so are quite safe, but you may not feel like undertaking more traveling than you have to.

Vacation Do's
- ☐ Talk to your doctor if you want to go away for longer than a month at any stage of your pregnancy.
- ☐ Get the name of a doctor in the place where you're going in case of emergency.
- ☐ Check with the doctor that you are allowed to have any vaccinations you may need.
- ☐ Work out a timetable allowing for delays. You won't feel like rushing.
- ☐ Ask the airline if they require a doctor's letter stating that you are fit to fly, especially if you are over thirty weeks pregnant. Most airlines will not let you fly after 36 weeks.
- ☐ Travel by train rather than by car for long distances – it's more comfortable.
- ☐ When on a long journey, try to stop and walk about every one or two hours.

Vacation Don't's
- ☐ Don't travel unless absolutely necessary in the first three months if you have had bleeding early in pregnancy or a previous miscarriage.
- ☐ Don't take drugs to prevent sea or air sickness without consulting your doctor.
- ☐ Don't travel far during the last six weeks and stay fairly close to home in the last four.
- ☐ Don't undertake long car journeys (three hours or more) unless accompanied by another driver.
- ☐ Don't eat too much unfamiliar food abroad, especially if highly spiced, and drink bottled, not local water.
- ☐ Don't travel anywhere too hot as you feel hotter naturally as pregnancy progresses.
- ☐ Don't go on a sports vacation. Riding, skiing, climbing and deep-sea diving can all wait.

Week 16

Month: Dates:

MON

TUES

WED

THURS

FRI

SAT

SUN

Notes

■ YOU AND YOUR DEVELOPING BABY

You If you have already had children you may well feel the first movements of the fetus, called 'quickening', about now. It is a sort of bubbling, fluttering sensation in your stomach.

Baby He is moving vigorously although his movements are rarely felt at this stage in a first pregnancy. However, if this is your second baby you may begin to feel him kick. His head is still quite large in comparison to his body size, but his body is catching up. His face is becoming more human, although his chin is still small and his mouth wide. His eyes are enormous, closed and spaced wide apart.

A fine downy hair (lanugo) appears all over your baby's body and face which is thought to keep him at the right temperature. Most of it will disappear before birth although sometimes a little hair is left which falls out later.

The external genital organs have now developed enough for your baby's sex to be detectable by ultrasound, although your untrained eye will probably not be able to see them.

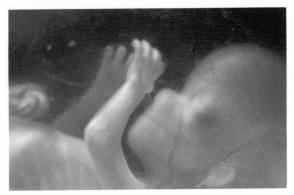

Your baby's skin is developing. It is transparent, but looks red because the blood vessels can be seen through it.

■ **DON'T FORGET** Make a note of the date when you first feel your baby move inside you.

Ultrasound scan

Your doctor may recommend that you have an ultrasound scan, or sonogram, in a hospital or, if he has the equipment, in his office. It may be interesting for your partner to be there with you.

An ultrasound is the modern equivalent of an X-ray and is at present considered much safer. It works by using sound waves to build up a photographic picture of your baby in the uterus. It can be used at any stage during pregnancy. If you are unsure about having a scan, talk to your doctor about it.

The scan will show you the outline of your baby's head and body on a screen and you will probaby see his backbone wriggling around like a sardine. Ask for the picture to be explained if you can't tell what's what.

What the scan tells you

☐ It determines how old your baby is, which is useful if you are unsure about the date of your last period. If done early in pregnancy this is accurate to within one week.

☐ It measures your baby to check that growth is proceeding normally.

☐ It picks up any visible abnormalities such as brain, head, spine or kidney conditions.

☐ It locates the position of the placenta and its condition.

☐ From around Week 9 an ultrasound scan will be able to detect whether or not you are expecting twins, so be prepared! If you are, you will receive special care and advice during pregnancy.

☐ It detects any growths in you that might make delivery difficult, such as fibroids.

☐ It finds the exact position of your baby and placenta before an amniocentesis is performed (see Week 17).

See Week 17 for Amniocentesis

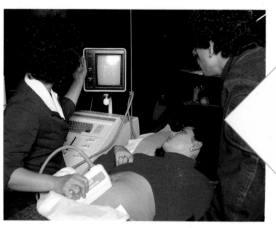

Having a scan
For your ultrasound examination, you lie on a bed and your bare abdomen is smeared with a jelly before the scanning machine is passed over it. The scan is painless (the only requirement being that you have a full bladder) and the results appear immediately on a television screen.

Twins
If you discover that you are expecting twins, you will have to take even greater care of yourself as you will probably get more tired and possibly feel more nauseous. You should take particular care with your diet. You will also have to plan well ahead to organize two sets of clothes and some equipment.

The average duration of a twin pregnancy is 36–38 weeks, so you will need to prepare yourself for labor, and have your hospital bag packed earlier. It would be worth reading a book on the subject and contacting a local Mothers of Twins Club (see Useful Addresses, p. 93).

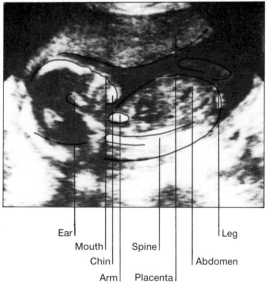

Ear
Mouth
Chin
Arm
Spine
Placenta
Leg
Abdomen

Week 17

Month: Dates:

MON

I think I might of felt the baby move 3/3/9?

TUES

WED

THURS

FRI

SAT

SUN

Notes

YOU AND YOUR DEVELOPING BABY

You You may find you are getting some pregnancy problems (see Weeks 11 and 12), such as a blocked nose or an increase in vaginal discharge or that you are sweating more than usual. The sweating is caused by the extra blood circulating in your system and may also make you feel hotter and your cheeks look rosier. All these common symptoms of pregnancy will vanish soon after delivery.

Your uterus is expanding quickly; you should now be able to feel the top of it roughly halfway between your pubic bone and your navel (see Week 20). You will probably have begun to look pregnant too. To reduce the possibility of back pain and discomfort later on, take steps to improve your posture (see Week 31).

Baby He can now hear sounds outside your body, which may make him jump. All his limbs are fully formed, as well as his skin and muscles. The chest muscles are starting to make movements similar to those that will be used in respiration. All his joints are able to move and about now you should begin to feel his movements. Tiny fingernails and toenails are beginning to appear.

Your baby measures approximately 7⅛in and now weighs more than the placenta.

DON'T FORGET Note the date when you first feel your baby moving.

Amniocentesis

Amniocentesis is a test carried out to detect certain abnormalities in the fetus. It has to be done at sixteen to eighteen weeks of pregnancy. A sample of the amniotic fluid which surrounds your baby is drawn out and tested for chromosomal abnormalities, such as Down's syndrome, and congenital abnormalities, such as spina bifida.

An ultrasound scan (see Week 16) is always done before the amniocentesis to check the position of the baby and the placenta so that neither is damaged by the needle. However, there is a small chance of an amniocentesis resulting in a miscarriage, so this test is not done on every expectant mother. Talk to your doctor if you are worried.

You have to wait about four weeks for the result of the test, which can be stressful. If any abnormality is discovered, you will be given the choice of continuing with your pregnancy or terminating it. You may feel there is no point in having an amniocentesis if abortion is against your principles, no matter what is wrong with your child.

Amniocentesis is offered to:

☐ Older women (over 35) for whom there is a higher risk of having a baby with Down's syndrome.

☐ Women who have a family history of Down's syndrome, spina bifida, hemophilia or muscular dystrophy.

☐ Women whose blood sample has shown a raised alpha-fetoprotein level, suggesting a spina bifida baby.

☐ Women who have already had a handicapped child.

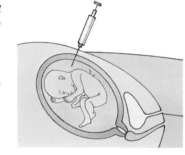

A needle is put through the wall of your abdomen to draw out a sample of amniotic fluid. The fluid is then tested for certain abnormalities.

See Weeks 21 and 22 for Keeping Fit

Pelvic floor exercises

Learning to contract and release your pelvic floor muscles efficiently will help you during labor by making you supple for the birth of your baby. It will also help prevent piles, incontinence and prolapse of your uterus. To see how efficient your pelvic muscles are, the next time you pass urine try to stop in mid-stream, hold for a few seconds and then relax.

Start exercising gradually. You can do pelvic floor exercises lying, sitting or standing. Imagine that your pelvic floor area is a lift going up. Contract it a little until you reach the first floor. Hold it there, then take it to the second floor and so on, until your muscles are fully contracted. Hold them for a count of six. Then release them gradually, floor by floor, until you have reached

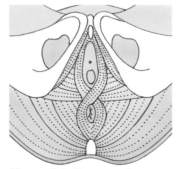

Your pelvic floor muscles are between your legs, forming a figure-8 around your front and back passages. They contract spontaneously during sexual intercourse.

the ground floor. Now push your pelvic floor downwards or away from you, as if you were blowing a candle out with your vagina and pant with your mouth open, slowly and deeply. This is the position your pelvic floor should be in when your baby's head is being born.

Rest and then repeat the above exercise six times, making sure that you are not holding your breath, tightening your shoulders or pulling in your stomach. The rest of your body should always be totally relaxed. If you do the above exercise four times after every visit to the toilet you will soon find you can hold your muscles firmly for a count of nine or ten.

Week 18

Month: Dates:

MON

TUES

WED

THURS

FRI

SAT

SUN

Notes

You If this is your first pregnancy, it is about now that you will probably feel your baby move for the first time. It's an exciting experience and a day you probably won't ever forget.

If you have flat or "inverted" (turned in) nipples, it could be a problem in later breast-feeding simply because there is little, if anything, for your baby to latch on to. It may help to massage your nipples several times a day, or you may be offered plastic breast shields to wear for a few hours a day. Most nipple problems, however, will be quickly remedied by a hungry baby.

Baby Your baby is now beginning to test his reflexes. He is kicking and punching with his well-formed arms and legs and possibly sucking his thumb as well. He is also twisting, turning and wriggling about. Inside his developing lungs tiny air sacs, called alveoli, are starting to form.

Your baby measures about 8in in length this week and is moving about much of the time.

Pregnancy wardrobe

During early pregnancy you may feel you want to attract attention to yourself – to wear bright red and announce to the world that you are expecting a baby. By the end of your pregnancy you will probably have found one or two outfits in which you feel comfortable and which you will want to wear day in, day out.

About now is a good time to go shopping for maternity wear. Earlier than this you may find it depressing seeing those skirts with added flaps and expandable waists: you don't want to imagine the size you will become. Once you've bought some maternity clothes, keep them in the closet for as long as you can and wear them only once they have become necessary, otherwise you'll get bored with them too soon – and so will your partner. It makes sense to buy some clothes for this intermediate stage of pregnancy that you can also wear while breast-feeding after the birth, i.e. with a front-opening. But make sure you have one or two outfits you feel good in: it's very important for your morale.

Dressing for a winter pregnancy is quite different from dressing for a summer one. In summer you will feel very hot but even in winter you won't feel the cold as much as usual: keep to lightweight natural fibers where possible (worn in layers in winter) and wash them often. Keep clothes loose-fitting – around your armholes as well as your waist.

Draw attention to your face and away from your belly with scarves, bows, collars and sailor's revers. Or draw the eye upward with bright lipstick, beautiful earrings or a hat.

Dresses Pinafores and smock-style dresses can be worn right through your pregnancy. Don't buy dresses with a tight bodice – you won't want your breasts to be restricted. Dresses with a dropped waist can look good but avoid styles with a seam at the waist: good though they may look around Week 19, they can be unflattering in Week 30.

Shoes Choose shoes that support your feet. Wear the same height of heel throughout your pregnancy: you will find it easiest to stand correctly if your heels are about 1in high. Avoid high heels: they can throw your weight forward and lead to backache. A long shoe horn will help you to put shoes on in late pregnancy.

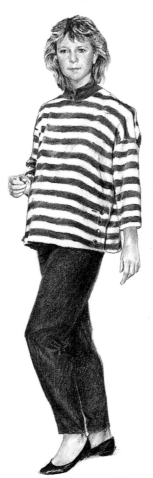

Coats Invest in a tent-shaped lightweight raincoat (or a cycling cloak, poncho or shawl), and wear it with layers of clothing. An ordinary coat left unbuttoned can look messy.

Underwear Wear cotton, not nylon, underwear if possible and make sure it is not too tight. Bikini briefs fit best under your belly. Use a lightweight maternity girdle if you feel you need support for your stomach. Wear a support bra from about Week 10 of your pregnancy.

Do not wear garters, elastic-top stockings or tight knee socks: they constrict the legs and can cause varicose veins. Wear support pantyhose if you have varicose veins.

Pants Always buy pants with an expandable waist. Jogging pants are comfortable – wear a large shirt, sweatshirt or T-shirt over them to cover your bottom. Dungarees and jumpsuits can be practical but are not always very flattering.

41

Week 19

Month: Dates:

MON

TUES

WED

THURS

FRI

SAT

SUN

Notes

You You are probably feeling a lot better and happier these days, especially once your baby's kicking has given you tangible proof of his presence. Share your baby's movements with your partner as soon as you can, though he may not be able to feel them as yet.

You will almost certainly have started to look pregnant now. In planning your maternity wardrobe, remember that you have a good few months to go and that the weather will probably not be the same when you are enormous as it is now. You may tire of your pregnancy clothes if you start wearing them too soon.

Baby This week buds for permanent teeth begin forming behind those that have already developed for the milk teeth. By now your child is drinking a considerable quantity of amniotic fluid each day. At the same time, his stomach is starting to secrete gastric juices, which will help him absorb the fluid. After absorption the fluid is filtered by his kidneys and excreted back into the amniotic sac.

Your baby now measures approximately 9in and a first-time mother may feel him move around now.

Vitamins and minerals

Ideally, your vitamin and mineral intake will come from food (see Week 3) but some women may need additional supplements. Such cases include:

☐ Women pregnant during adolescence (they are still growing themselves).

☐ Women who are underweight or run-down or who were eating an unbalanced diet when they became pregnant.

☐ Women who were overweight when they became pregnant.

☐ Women on a strict diet, such as vegetarians and macrobiotics.

☐ Women who are allergic to certain vital foods, such as cow's milk or wheat.

☐ Women who have previously lost a baby from miscarriage or stillbirth.

☐ Women who have had three pregnancies in the last two years.

☐ Women suffering from chronic diseases for which they take continuous medication.

☐ Women who have a multiple pregnancy.

☐ Women who have to work particularly hard or who are under a lot of stress.

☐ Women who smoke, drink or take drugs.

Unless indicated, there is no need to take increased amounts of the following vitamins during pregnancy.

See Week 3 for Healthy Eating

Vitamins

Vitamin A for resistance to infection, relief of allergies or acne, good vision, formation of tooth enamel, hair and fingernails.

☐ Dairy products, oily fish, liver, cooked carrots, apricots, tomatoes and greens.

B Vitamins (1, 2, 3, 5, 6 and 12) for eye and skin problems, nervousness, constipation, lack of energy; milk production, digestion, infection, bleeding gums, development of healthy red blood cells.

☐ Whole grains, wheatgerm (don't overcook), beans, nuts, liver, pork, egg yolk, brewer's yeast, milk, cheese, mushrooms, potatoes, bananas, green vegetables, oily fish, wholewheat bread, brown rice.

Vitamin C for absorption of iron, strong and healthy tissues, resistance to infection, building a strong placenta and healing fractures and wounds. May be prescribed during pregnancy to help absorb iron.

☐ Citrus fruits, berry fruits, green, red and yellow raw vegetables, potatoes.

Vitamin D for absorption of calcium and phosphorus, and building strong bones.

☐ Found in oily fish, dairy products, liver – and sunlight on the skin.

Vitamin E for improved circulation, varicose veins, piles and hormone production.

☐ Most foods, especially wheatgerm, eggs.

Vitamin K Helps your blood to clot (useful after a difficult delivery).

☐ Green vegetables and alfalfa sprouts.

Folic acid For development of your baby's central nervous system, blood formation, prevention of spina bifida and other malformations. Twice the normal amount is needed during pregnancy and is often prescribed at the same time as iron, after Week 14.

☐ Raw leafy vegetables, walnuts, liver.

Minerals

Calcium Needed for the development of strong bones and teeth in your baby. It also enables your blood to clot and your muscles to work smoothly. You need almost twice as much calcium during pregnancy and breast-feeding, especially in the first four months of pregnancy. Vitamin D is essential for your body to absorb calcium efficiently.

☐ Leafy vegetables, turnips, cauliflower, fish, oranges, raspberries, blackberries, dairy foods, whole grains, beans and nuts.

Iron Needed in the formation of hemoglobin for your increased number of red blood cells. Vitamin C helps your body absorb iron. You need about twice as much iron during pregnancy as you do normally. If you are taking antacid medicines for indigestion you may need extra iron (ask your doctor).

☐ Liver, egg yolk, herring, sardines, whole grains, beans, dark green leaf vegetables, raisins, prunes, nuts, dark molasses, brewer's yeast.

Salt Needed in pregnancy because the salt in your blood is diluted by increased body fluids.

Week 20

Month:
February

Dates:
29

MON

TUES

WED

* THURS

FRI

SAT

SUN

Notes

YOU AND YOUR DEVELOPING BABY

You Your uterus is beginning to enlarge more rapidly from now on; it presses up against your lungs and pushes your stomach outwards so you begin to look more pregnant. You should be able to feel your uterus just under your navel. Your navel may be starting to flatten or pop out – it will stay that way until after delivery.

Baby Your baby is growing rapidly in both weight and length and now measures approximately 10in which is roughly half of what the average baby measures at birth. His weight is around 12oz. His growth will soon slow down a little. His muscles are increasing in strength and active movements can now be felt. They may feel like light flutters or like bubbles bursting against your abdomen.

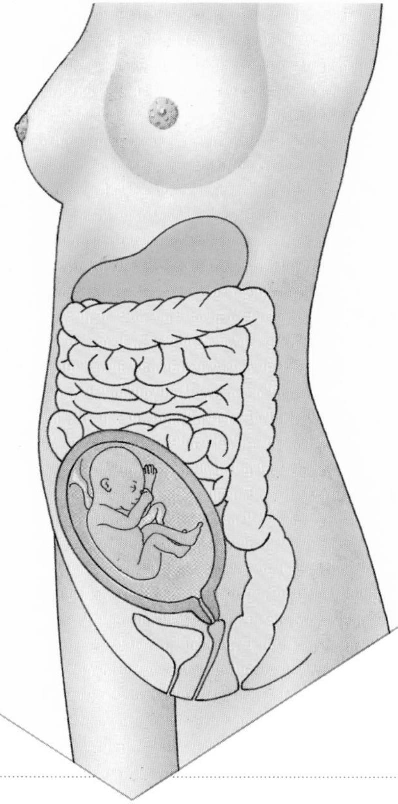

Height of fundus

The fundus is the top of your uterus and its height is a gauge used by your doctor to see how far advanced your pregnancy is. It is normally measured in centimeters from your pubic bone.

In order to accommodate your growing baby your uterus will have to increase its volume about 1,000-fold during pregnancy and, as it does, it will take up the space of other organs. This can lead to some of the problems of later pregnancy, such as breathlessness, constipation, heartburn and frequency of urination.

On average a non-pregnant uterus is roughly the size of a tangerine. It measures approximately 7cm (2¾in) in length, 5cm (2in) in width and is over 2.5cm (1in) thick. By six weeks it is the size of an apple and two weeks later that of an orange. By twelve weeks the uterus is the size of a grapefruit and by Week 14 it will look like a small melon. At full term it can measure as much as 38cm (15in) in length, 25.5cm (10in) in width and 20cm (8in) from front to back. The weight of the uterus itself increases during pregnancy by approximately twenty times, from a pre-pregnant weight of 40g (2oz) to almost 800g (2lb) at its heaviest, immediately after pregnancy.

With your first child, a phenomenon called "lightening" may occur after Week 36 which means that your baby drops slightly and engages in your pelvis. Your fundus thus descends a little even though your uterus has not shrunk – this will put pressure on your groin and pelvis. With a second or subsequent baby, this may not happen until the onset of labor.

Although your uterus is expanding throughout your pregnancy, you will probably only notice it after Week 12 when it becomes too large to stay hidden in your pelvis. From then on it enlarges at a regular rate until Week 36 when it reaches to just below your breastbone. This may make it awkward to breathe and you may feel a jabbing pain in your ribcage.

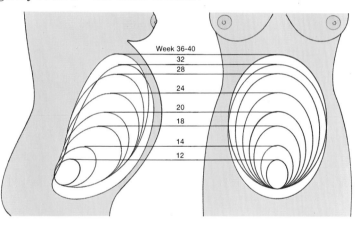

Week 36-40
32
28
24
20
18
14
12

Pre-eclampsia

Pre-eclampsia is also known as toxemia. It is a possible condition of later pregnancy involving raised blood pressure and protein in your urine; it rarely occurs before Week 20. It usually develops slowly and there is a risk to both you and your unborn baby if it goes unnoticed. This is one of the reasons why it is important to go for regular prenatal visits at which your blood pressure and urine are tested. Look out for the signs and alert your doctor if you notice any of them.

It is best to prevent pre-eclampsia, but if it develops and is severe you may have to go to the hospital for bedrest, sedation and monitoring of the kidney function and blood pressure. It usually improves under these conditions and will certainly disappear completely once your baby is born.

What the doctor will be looking out for:
- [ ] swelling of the feet, ankles, face and hands due to fluid retention;
- [ ] raised blood pressure;
- [ ] protein in your urine (this is why you take a urine sample to the hospital every visit);
- [ ] excessive weight gain.

Week 21

Month: _march_   Dates: _7_

MON

TUES

WED

✗ THURS

FRI

SAT

SUN

Notes

You By the end of this week you should be able to feel the top of your womb about level with your navel. Around now you will probably be starting to feel energetic, healthy and very positive – in short, better than you have ever felt before. You may notice that you are beginning to get a lot done. Remember to rest even if you don't feel like it. You may be feeling constantly hungry as well. During the next ten weeks is when you put on about half of the weight you gain during pregnancy (see Week 25) so watch what you eat. Eat well – but not for two.

Baby Around now your baby's skin becomes opaque. White blood cells are starting to be manufactured, which play an important part in fighting disease and infection. Your child's tongue is now fully developed, and, if female, her internal organs of reproduction – the vagina and the womb – have formed. His legs are now in proportion with the rest of his body and his movements are becoming increasingly sophisticated.

Your baby has been growing steadily and now weighs around 1lb and measures about 11in in length.

Keeping fit/1

Try and keep active during pregnancy. Not only will it stand you in good stead during your demanding labor but it means you will be less likely to stiffen up as your pregnancy progresses. It will also help you to regain your normal shape more quickly after delivery.

Check with your doctor before exercising during the first three months if you have had a previous miscarriage or are experiencing any complications with this pregnancy. Do all exercises slowly; carry them out rhythmically – never quickly or jerkily – and relax for a minute or two after completing each one.

Never strain yourself and don't exercise until you drop or are in pain. Remember that you are having a baby, not training for the Olympics. Never do sit-ups or raise both legs simultaneously while lying down when you are pregnant. Either can damage your abdominal muscles and strain your back.

Keep breathing at a controlled pace and try to relax the parts of your body which are not being exercised. Arrange pillows where necessary to keep comfortable and always get up from the floor by rolling on to your side and using your arms to push you up. After you have carried out your exercises, lie on your back and rest for a few minutes.

Below are some exercises for you to do gently. Further exercises, to strengthen your back, breast muscles and pelvic muscles, are given in Week 22.

See Week 17 for Pelvic Floor Exercises

See Week 31 for Good Posture

Hip stretching
Sit upright on the floor with your back straight (or lean against a wall).
1. With the soles of your feet together, and your heels as near to your body as possible, gently push your knees towards the floor. If this is difficult, push one knee first and then the other.
2. Keeping your legs flat on the floor, move them as far apart as you can. You should feel your groin stretching. ▽

Circulation in legs
1. Lie on your back with a pillow under your knees to prevent back strain. Lift your left leg a little way off the ground and, keeping your knees straight, rotate your left ankle, first clockwise, then anti-clockwise, six times. Repeat with your right ankle.
2. Stand up and, keeping your left foot flat on the ground and your left leg straight, tiptoe on to your right foot. Then, bending your left knee and straightening your right leg, with your right foot now flat on the ground, tiptoe on to your left foot. Do this gentle exercise whenever you have to stand for any length of time.

Stomach muscles (abdominal wall)
1. Lie on your back with your knees bent and your feet flat on the floor. Have a pillow under your head and shoulders. Tighten your stomach muscles so that your abdomen is gently pulled down towards your back. Hold for three seconds, then relax slowly. (This exercise is also good for regaining your figure after birth.)
2. Keeping the small of your back pressed down, slowly stretch both legs until they are straight. Draw one knee back up, and then the other, without lifting the small of your back off the floor. If your back hurts at any point, stop. Otherwise repeat until you can do the exercise ten times. ▽

Week 22

Month:
march

Dates:
_14_

MON

TUES

WED

*THURS

FRI

SAT

SUN

Notes

You You will probably notice that your baby is developing a pattern of waking and sleeping and may well be at his most active while you are wanting to sleep. You may sometimes be able to feel him high in your stomach and sometimes low down near your pubis. At this stage his kicks are endearing, and still quite gentle; they may get fiercer!

You may find that you are bringing up small amounts of acid fluid; antacid tablets will help neutralize this. Your gums may bleed more than usual

Baby By the end of the fifth month vernix, a greasy, white, cheesy-looking substance, is beginning to form on your child's skin. Vernix is a mixture of sebum, from the sebaceous glands, and skin cells. It protects your baby's delicate, newly-formed skin from the possible damage of living in liquid for nine months and also against the increasing concentration of urine in the amniotic fluid. The vernix adheres to the lanugo all over the skin. Although most of the vernix will have disappeared before birth, some is left to lubricate your baby's passage along the birth canal during delivery and is one reason why a newborn baby is so slippery and difficult to handle.

Your baby has now grown to about 11½in long and weighs about 1lb 2oz.

DON'T FORGET Go and see your dentist if you haven't already.

48

Keeping fit/2

Below are some more exercises for you to do gently (read Week 21 before starting these). If you can't face even these, do at least go for a daily walk or a swim.

Squatting makes your pelvic joints more flexible and stretches and strengthens thighs and back muscles. It can also relieve back pain.

Swimming

Start to use the local pool: swimming is wonderful exercise for pregnancy. Even if you can't swim you can exercise by holding on to the side of the pool, with your back to the wall, and cycling in the water, or by facing the side of the pool and swaying gently from side to side.

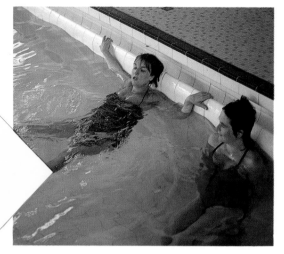

See Week 31 for Good Posture

Squatting

1. Full squats Keeping your back straight, and legs apart, squat down low. Distribute your weight evenly between heels and toes. To further stretch, press elbows against inner thighs.

2. Half squats Hold on to a chair and place your right foot in front of your left. Point your right knee slightly out and slowly bend both knees. Keep your bottom tucked in and back straight. Stand up slowly, then repeat with the other leg in front.

Back strengthening

1. Pelvic rock Lie on your back with your feet together, flat on the floor, and knees slightly bent. Place a hand under the hollow of your back. Using your stomach muscles, press your spine against the floor until your back is flat. Relax and repeat.

2. The cat Get on all fours with your hands and knees apart. Arch your back gently and push your head down so you feel a stretch from neck to tail. Now raise your head as you relax your back to its normal position. Repeat once.

Breast muscles

Sit cross-legged on the floor with your back straight. Bend your arms and grip your left wrist with your right hand and vice versa. Breathe in and blow out once. Now breathe in, hold your breath and push your shoulders and ribcage down. Tip your chin gently on to your chest and push your arm muscles towards your elbows ten times. Then raise your head and blow out slowly. Repeat once. If you find you can't hold your breath for so long, build up to it slowly.

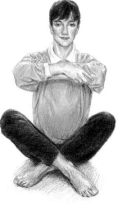

Week 23

Month: _March_

MON

TUES

WED

*THURS

FRI

SAT

SUN

Notes

YOU AND YOUR DEVELOPING BABY

You You may have already noticed a painless, though uncomfortable, hardening of your stomach which occurs roughly every twenty minutes and lasts for twenty seconds. You may have thought it was your baby's foot or bottom pushing your stomach, but this is a "Braxton Hicks" uterine contraction; they occur all the way through pregnancy, although they are not usually noticeable before this stage. They help your uterus grow and ensure a good circulation of blood through your uterine vessels.

You may also sometimes get a stitch-like pain down the side of your stomach, which is your uterine muscle stretching. Have a rest and the pain will go.

Baby Your baby is now moving vigorously, often in response to touch and sound. A loud noise nearby may make him jump and kick. He is also swallowing small amounts of amniotic fluid and passing tiny amounts of urine back into it. Sometimes he may get hiccups and you can feel the jerk of each hiccup.

His heartbeat can now be heard through a stethoscope. Your partner may even be able to hear it by putting his ear to your tummy, but he has to find the right place and the room has to be quiet.

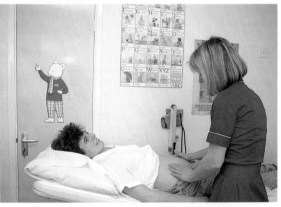

The midwife may have to move the baby into a position where his heartbeat can be heard.

The father's role

Your partner is no doubt as pleased as you are about your pregnancy and the future baby. He will also be concerned, although his anxieties may well be different from yours. He may worry about how your relationship will change, about how his life will be disrupted and about whether he is going to be able to support you both financially (especially if you are giving up work). It may also be difficult at first for him to realize that a baby is really there; it can feel strange being so closely involved and yet in a sense so removed.

Include him as much as possible, and make him feel proud – after all, it is his baby

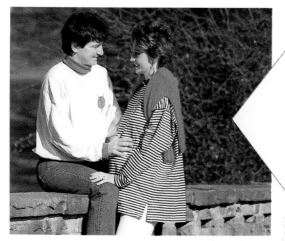

too. Let him feel the baby kicking, invite him along to hospital appointments, prenatal classes and, of course, the birth – but don't be upset if he feels he doesn't want to come. If he doesn't attend, let him know all you've been told at the hospital or at classes. But try not to become a pregnancy bore unless you feel he is really interested. If it is your first child, try and do as much together now as you can, whether it's reading the papers in bed in the morning, going to the movies regularly or going away on vacation.

Explain to your partner how you are feeling, because your emotions will be changing a lot more than usual. Make sure you apologize if you find yourself snapping at him. Try and get him to help out if you are

feeling sick or too tired to do anything – especially during the first and the last three months. If you have other children, he can play a very important part in your pregnancy (see Week 14).

Your partner may feel jealous both of the coming child and of your ability to nurture new life within you. He may also dislike being the supporting actor rather than the star and may feel he is only peripherally helpful. Partners need both physical and mental reassurance. Even if you don't feel like sex, cuddle and caress him, and try not to let the ten pillows that surround your body in bed every night get in between you too much! Try and talk to your partner about his emotions and worries, even if you feel more like concentrating on yourself.

See Week 38 for Fathers in Labor

See Weeks 6 and 24 for Sex during Pregnancy

To fathers

Be positive and appreciative: always let your partner know she is doing her best. Try to be sympathetic and supportive – always show her you love her and help her where you can. If at times you feel left out, rest assured that what you are sharing will bond the two of you closer together all your lives. Read all you can about pregnancy and childbirth, and prepare yourself for adjustments afterwards.

Practical checklist for fathers

☐ Do you know the quickest route to the hospital, the correct entrance and where you can park?

☐ Have you visited the hospital beforehand to see where the delivery rooms, canteen and wards are?

☐ Have you put a blanket and some cushions in the car?

☐ Do you know what the signs of labor are? (See Week 37)

☐ Have you discussed what your partner feels about pain relief? (See Week 35)

☐ If you want to attend the birth, are you as knowledgeable about it as your partner?

☐ Are the relevant phone numbers displayed by the phone? (See Week 37)

Week 24

Month: _march_

Dates: 28

MON

TUES

WED

✱THURS

FRI

SAT

SUN

Notes

You You may begin to put on weight fairly rapidly about now and your feet will probably start to feel the strain. Check that your shoes are comfortable and give you enough support; go barefoot at home if you feel like it. Rest with your feet up – preferably above your heart – whenever possible.

If you are finding your job more and more exhausting try to arrange to leave work, or to work part-time, from early in the third trimester (from Week 28 on) if your employer agrees.

Baby Your baby is still rather thin and his skin quite wrinkled because he has not yet laid down deposits of fat, but he is growing lengthwise. His arms and legs now have a normal amount of muscle and they are moving vigorously. Creases are appearing on his palms and fingertips.

If he was delivered this week his vital organs are sufficiently developed for him to be able to survive for a short time, but his lungs are not quite mature enough for him to be able to live for long outside your uterus.

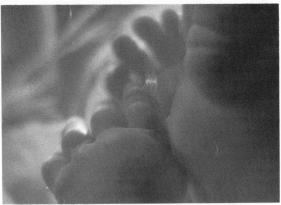

Your baby's hands are active at this time. This muscular coordination is sufficiently developed for him to suck his thumb!

Problems of later pregnancy

Some minor problems, or discomforts, start in early pregnancy and continue until the last few months (see Weeks 11 and 12). Others only begin towards, or during, the final trimester. You may of course experience few, or none, of them.

Backache See Week 31
Breathlessness From about Week 30 you might find

Discomfort in bed
This could be due to indigestion or heartburn, or to pressure from your enlarged uterus. If your mattress is not firm, place a board under it. Distribute pillows under different parts of your body until you get comfortable. Lying on your right side may be most comfortable (see Week 31).

---

breathing difficult, due to pressure on your diaphragm from your growing uterus. It will become easier once your baby's head has engaged. Remember to sit up or stand as straight as possible, and prop a few pillows under your head and shoulders in bed. If you have chest pain or swelling, consult your doctor.

Incontinence You may leak a little urine when you cough, laugh or bend down. This could be due to your enlarged uterus pressing on your bladder, or to weak pelvic floor muscles (see Week 17). Empty your bladder often and avoid lifting anything heavy; exercise your pelvic floor.

Indigestion and heartburn
Some of the foods you normally enjoy may give you indigestion. If you can work out what they are, avoid them. Eat smaller meals and sit up straight when eating to take the pressure off your stomach.

Heartburn is a burning pain in the lower part of your chest, throat, back of your mouth or stomach, often accompanied by the regurgitation of sour fluid. It is caused by the relaxation of a stomach valve, allowing acid to pass into the tube.

Sleep with your shoulders well propped up, or even with telephone directories under the head end of your bed. A glass of milk, or spring or soda water, before sleeping may help. Don't sit slumped in a chair and try not to bend down, putting your head below your chest; avoid rich, fried or spicy foods; and wear clothes that are loose at the waist. If the problem gets serious, see your doctor.

Nausea Nausea towards the end of pregnancy may be due to the pressure of your uterus on your stomach. Eat small, frequent meals. (See Week 7)

Pelvic discomfort You may develop pain around your pubic area, or in your groin and down the inside of your thighs. This could be caused by your baby's head pressing on nerves, or by your pelvic joints softening in preparation for labor. Don't stand or sit for long periods and avoid violent exercise. Rest frequently and take the occasional Tylenol tablet if the pain gets too uncomfortable.

"Pins and needles" This is due to the increase in body fluid exerting pressure on your

nerves and tendons. Hold your hands above your head and wriggle your fingers.

Rib pain After about Week 30, when the top of the uterus is high, you may feel a pain just below your breasts. You will feel most comfortable sitting on a straight chair or lying down flat. Stretch upwards to lift your ribcage off your uterus.

Swelling of legs, ankles, fingers (edema) Edema is an increase in fluid retention in your body, especially in the lower limbs. This is due to the pressure of the uterus on the vessels that return blood from the lower parts of your body to the heart. You may notice your shoes feeling tight, your ankles becoming wrinkled and your rings not fitting. Mention this to your doctor in case it is a sign of pre-eclampsia (see Week 20). Avoid standing, and rest on your bed for an hour or two a day, with your feet raised above your heart. It may help to wear maternity support tights. Avoid garters or tight socks or shoes.

Sex in later pregnancy
The classic missionary position (with the man on top) is uncomfortable in the later stages. But this is no reason to give up sex. Try "the spoons" position, both facing the same way – you lying on your side with your partner close behind you. Or you can kneel or crouch so your partner can enter you from behind. Or find ways other than penetration to have sex.

See Week 6 for Your Relationship

See Weeks 11 and 12 for Common Problems

Week 25

Month: *april* Dates: *4*

MON

TUES

WED

✗THURS

FRI

SAT

SUN

Notes

You Around now is the best time in pregnancy for many women. Make the most of it. You may find that you are looking flushed and rosy-cheeked with the increase in blood circulation underneath your skin. You should also be feeling happy and contented; if you are not, try and talk about it to your partner, friends and your doctor.

The minus side is that you may be experiencing some of the problems of pregnancy, such as backache, cramps and a desire to urinate more often.

Your heart and lungs are now doing fifty per cent more work than usual and you will find that you are sweating more because of your raised body fluid levels.

Baby Your baby's bone centers are beginning to harden. From now on he is growing slowly and steadily, his body growing at a faster pace to catch up with the size of his head. He will be fattening out as well, so that his eyes seem less hollow in his head. During the last seven days he will have grown just under ½in and gained just over 3oz in weight.

Growing at a steady pace, your baby now measures about 1ft 2in and weighs around 1lb 4oz.

54

Weight gain in pregnancy

At one stage it was thought that pregnant women should "eat for two". Then opinions changed and women were led to believe that they should try not to gain weight during pregnancy as it would stay with them forever. Today, studies show that underweight women are probably at greater risk of bearing low-birthweight babies and that a steady weight gain is desirable.

You will be weighed each time you go to the doctor's, partly to show that your baby is growing normally and partly to check on your own health: a sudden change up or down in weight could signify problems. If you are putting on too much weight it could indicate a condition of pre-eclampsia (see Week 20). Dieting and cutting down on fluids will not help, so continue to eat well.

The diagram below shows how your weight gain is made up. However much weight you put on during pregnancy, you will gain roughly a quarter of the total between Weeks 12 and 20, half between Weeks 20 and 30 and the last quarter between Weeks 30 and 38. If you find your weight shooting up at the end, this is probably due to water retention, so don't worry. You will lose it all after your baby is born, although it follows that the less weight you put on, the easier this will be lost.

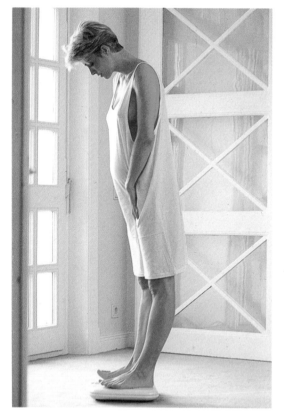

See Week 3 for Healthy Eating

See Week 19 for Vitamins and Minerals

Most women gain about 30lb altogether during pregnancy and find that they are 7–14lb heavier after giving birth than before they became pregnant. The amount varies between individuals and in one woman from one pregnancy to the next.

One indication of how much superfluous fat you will be left with after the birth is to measure your upper thighs each week. Their circumference should stay the same throughout most of your pregnancy, as this is your own body fat, although towards the end of your pregnancy fluid retention may increase this measurement.

Remember that individual women gain weight at different rates. If you are worried about your weight, discuss it with your doctor; do not start dieting during pregnancy. You can do more harm to yourself and your baby by eating too little of the foods you need than by eating too much.

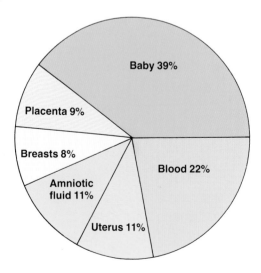

Pregnancy weight gain chart

55

Week 26

Month: april Dates: 11

MON

TUES

WED

*THURS

FRI

SAT

SUN

Notes

YOU AND YOUR DEVELOPING BABY

You Take advantage of your surplus energy and any spare time to start preparing for your child's arrival. If you think you're busy now, you'll certainly be busier later on! Get organized: make lists of anything you need to do around your home and any clothes and other equipment you need to buy.

If you haven't already, start to use the local swimming pool, go for a daily walk or do a regular regimen of exercises.

Baby The branches of your baby's lungs (the bronchi) are now developing, but his lungs will not be fully formed until after he is born. His head is growing faster than his body at this time and is now in better proportion to his body. Fat stores are beginning to accumulate.

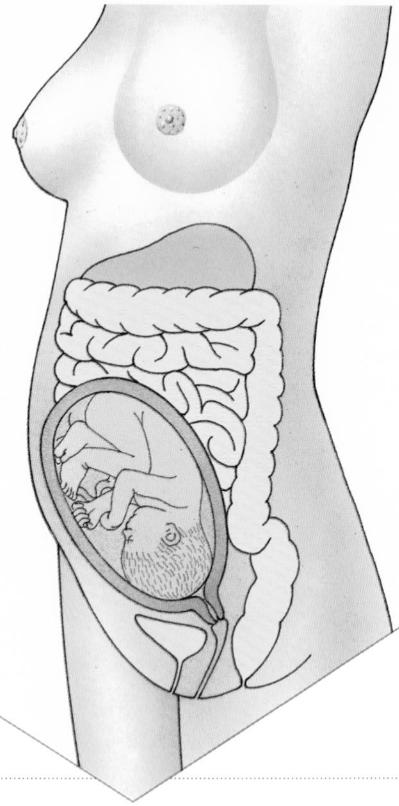

Preparing for baby

It is not essential that your baby has a room of his own: he can equally well share with older siblings or with you. If he's to share your bedroom it is a good idea to keep him in a separate corner so you will have some privacy. Put a well-shaded lamp in the baby's section so as not to wake your partner (unless he wants to help) when you have to change and feed your child in the night.

If he can have his own room, it's nice to make it bright and colorful and appealing for a child, but there is no need to spend a lot of money on baby equipment or on totally redecorating a room that has just been done. Your child will be happiest sleeping and playing in a room in which he can relax and enjoy himself – and that won't happen if you are worried about him ruining the decor. Remember that he will grow quickly and his requirements will constantly be changing. Whether you are preparing the baby's room from scratch or furnishing and adapting a room, there are several considerations to bear in mind.

Floors If you haven't yet laid a carpet, consider using non-slip vinyl (easy to clean), or else cork or carpet tiles so that you can replace the odd one rather than the whole carpet. Use non-slip polish on wooden floors and make sure there are no splinters. Small mats or rugs can be slippery, so avoid them or use a non-slip backing.

Furniture Furniture should be sufficiently heavy that it can't be pulled over. Paint any baby furniture that you inherit, such as crib or child's bed, with non-toxic paint (i.e. not lead-based) for safety. Bring in a low, comfortable chair (preferably without arms) with a straight back for feeding and put a small table or storage box at the side.

You will need drawer space for clothes and some storage space for diapers. Provided a chest of drawers is the right height, you could use the top of it as a changing place.

Heating It is important that your baby's room is kept warm by day and night in cold weather. Try to keep a constant temperature of about 68°F for the first few weeks. If you are using an approved, UL labeled space heater or heating stove in your child's bed-room, be sure to turn it off or turn low before going to bed. Wood stoves and fireplaces must be screened by a fixed guard with a small mesh. Rooms heated by kerosene heaters must be properly ventilated and heaters regularly serviced. Install a humidifier if the air gets too dry.

Lamps Overhead lighting is preferable: table lamps can be knocked over and electric wires tripped over. Cover sockets with special childproof covers. A dimmer switch or night-light allows you to check your baby without waking him up.

Walls Painted walls are easier to clean. Wallpaper should be washable and preferably have a pattern that doesn't show every fingerprint.

Windows Make sure windows (and doors) are draftproof or that your baby does not sleep too close to them. Windows should be fixed so that they cannot be opened far enough for him to fall out. Guard low windows with close-spaced vertical bars (removable in case of fire). Use a thick material for curtains or line them well to make sure they keep the light out. You can buy a special rubber-backed "blackout" lining material (which is in fact white).

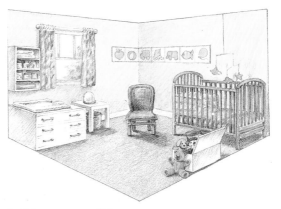

In this nursery, useful storage – shelves, chest of drawers and toy box – combine with colorful accessories – frieze and crib mobile – to make an attractive and practical room.

See Weeks 27 and 28 for Shopping for Equipment

See Week 32 for Getting Ready

See Week 33 for Shopping for Layette

Week 27

Month: april   Dates: 18

MON
april - 21 7 months 2002

TUES

WED

*THURS

FRI

SAT

SUN

Notes

YOU AND YOUR DEVELOPING BABY

You You are probably beginning to put on weight at a steady rate and may be aware that you are starting to get more tired. As you come to the end of your middle trimester, you may begin to experience a few of the minor problems commonly associated with later pregnancy (see Week 24).

You may notice quite regular Braxton Hicks contractions now, especially when walking. Try wearing a lightweight maternity corset if you feel it would help. Keep exercising. You should now be able to feel the top of your uterus about halfway between your navel and your breast bone.

Baby Around this week the membranes which formed your baby's eyelids part, and his eyelids open for the first time. His eyes are almost always blue or dark blue at this stage as the eye coloring is not fully developed until a few months after birth. Occasionally, however, a baby's eyes turn brown within only a few hours of him being born.

Your baby now weighs about 2lb and measures around 1ft 2in.

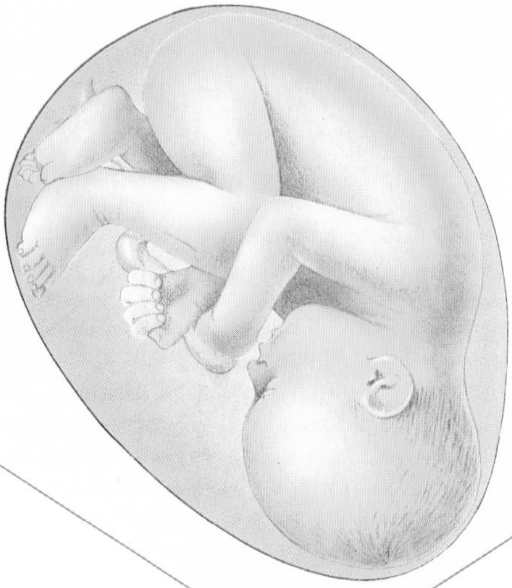

Shopping for equipment/1

It is a good idea to shop for equipment, and possibly baby clothes too, at this stage, while you still have the energy. You will probably feel too tired and uncomfortable for shopping in the later stages of pregnancy – and you will have no time at all once the baby is born! If you feel it is "tempting fate" to fill the house with baby things before he is even born, most stores will let you order major pieces of equipment now, provided you leave a deposit, and will deliver them to your home after the birth.

If this is your first baby it can be difficult to know exactly what you will need and the choice can be baffling. The suggestions below and in Week 28 will help you to make decisions. If this is your second or subsequent child, you probably already have most of the furniture and equipment you'll need. If you're buying new equipment, always make sure that it complies with government safety regulations.

Below is a list of major items of sleep equipment you might buy and the points to bear in mind when choosing them.

Crib You don't need a full-size crib at first but something smaller, such as a portable bassinet, portacrib, Moses basket or carriage.

If you borrow or inherit a used crib, check that the paint or varnish is non-toxic and that there are no splinters or sharp edges

anywhere. Check also that the gap between bars conforms with standards set by the Consumer Product Safety Commission. In choosing a new one, see that it's sturdy enough and that the sides are high enough to prevent a child climbing out. Choose one with a drop side or you'll have to stoop low to lift your baby in and out, but check that it has a safety catch to prevent him letting down the sides himself when he is older.

Crib mattress This needs to be firm and is best covered with plastic. It should fit the crib with no space around the edges.

Bedding You will need at least three bottom sheets. Fitted cotton or flannel sheets are cozy though they take longer to dry. Your baby won't use top sheets for the first few weeks as he will be wrapped in a shawl or light blanket. After that three nonfitted flannel sheets will be enough. He must not use a pillow for at least the first year, but he will need blankets or a blanket and quilt. Several light layers (preferably cotton cellular blankets) are warmer and more comfortable than one heavy one; avoid fringes which your baby may suck. You could use a washable duvet (and two duvet covers) instead.

Baby monitor This will let you hear the baby crying if you live in a large or noisy house. You can get one that has a battery-operated receiver that clips on to your belt so that you can take it from room to room.

See
Week 28 for
Shopping for
Equipment/2

See
Week 33 for
Shopping for
Layette

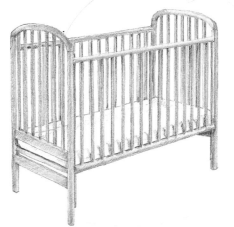

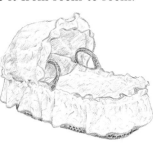

◁ *A useful feature in some cribs is an adjustable height mattress.*

A Moses basket makes a cozy first bed.▷

You can get spring interior crib mattresses (bottom) or ones made of foam with or without air vents. ▷

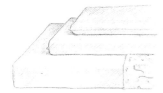

Week 28

MON

TUES

WED

*THURS

FRI

SAT

SUN

Notes

YOU AND YOUR DEVELOPING BABY

You Week 28 is the first week of your third and last trimester, which often seems the longest. Some of the minor problems of pregnancy, such as indigestion and cramps, may have become a part of life but be assured they will disappear after the birth. Get as much rest and sleep as possible and keep up your calcium intake by eating more milk, cheese or yogurt.

Baby At 28 weeks your baby is considered "viable", which means he is thought capable of sustaining separate and independent life if born. His lungs are reaching maturity and although he might have breathing problems and difficulty keeping himself warm if born, with modern special care facilities he has a chance of survival.

By now your baby is large enough for his position in your uterus to be assessed during an abdominal examination. He may be in the usual head downwards position or in a breech position (*see* Understanding your Medical Records, page 88).

Your baby now measures approximately 1ft 2½in and weighs roughly 2lb 3oz.

Shopping for equipment/2

Major items of equipment for transporting your baby are assessed below.

Carseat An approved safety carseat is essential. It is the safest way to transport an infant, and is a legal requirement in most states. There are many different models from which to choose. You should decide before you buy whether you want a carseat that can be easily taken in and out of the car, or one that remains in place for the duration of its use. For information and recommendations on carseats, contact your state's Highway Safety Program or the National Highway Traffic Safety Administration (see Useful Addresses, p. 93). Some communities have rental programs for approved safety seats; contact your local health department for details.

Carriage When choosing a carriage, check that it is light enough for you to push easily, that the handles are at a comfortable height and that the brakes can be operated without letting go of the handle. Make sure the hood goes up and down easily, that the wheels run smoothly (large wheels may be easier to push), that the mattress is firm and that a shopping tray can be fitted without interfering with the brakes. Make sure there are anchor points for a safety harness.

Carriage harness Buy one that is strong and washable and easy to fasten and unfasten.

Carriage net This will keep off insects.

Stroller Newborn babies shouldn't travel in upright or even semi-upright strollers as their back muscles are not strong enough to support them sitting up. Wait until your baby has grown out of the portable bassinet before buying a stroller, or buy one that will let him lie flat or that will take a portable bassinet clipped to the main frame.

Make sure the back is firm enough to give support. Are there built-in safety straps, or anchor points for your carriage harness? Check that it's light enough to carry easily and see how simple it is to fold with one hand – imagine holding a baby in the other. Make sure that the brakes lock and there are no sharp edges.

Baby carrier or sling Your baby will enjoy being held close to you and it leaves your hands free. Check that it has adjustable straps and a padded head support, preferably detachable for later.

Portable bassinet This may suit you better than a carriage if you are using the portable bassinet as your baby's bed, or taking it in the car. Make sure the handles are strong and well balanced and that it is light enough to carry. NOTE: It is very dangerous to hold a baby in your arms or transport a baby in a bassinet or basket in the car – even if it is secured with a seatbelt; an approved infant carseat is required.

See Week 27 for Shopping for Equipment/1

See Week 33 for Shopping for Layette

Equipment for transporting baby

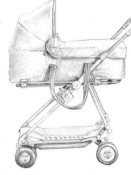 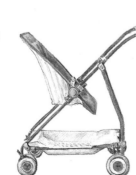 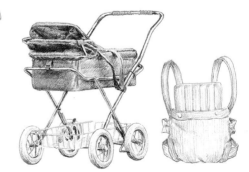 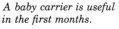 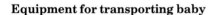

An all-in-one carriage with portable bassinet.

A multi-position stroller.

A portable bassinet and transporter.

A baby carrier is useful in the first months.

Week 29 96

Month:
may

Dates: 3

MON

TUES

WED ✳

THURS

✳ FRI

SAT

SUN

Notes

You By now you will probably be able to tell your baby's bottom from his knee. In the bath you may be able to watch him move from one side of your abdomen to another. 's hand movements are softer than his rather jerky kn and foot movements.

If you haven't already ne so, go for a swim. You will enjoy feeling much light r than you do normally. You may start needing to si down often and you probably won't feel like running a round. Start delegating some chores to your partner.

Baby Your baby has filled almost all the space in your uterus and his head is now more or less in proportion with his body. Although he may still be lying with his head up, within a few weeks he should have turned upside down and will then appear to fit more comfortably. He is growing at a weekly rate of just under ⅜in and now measures around 1ft 3in.

Your baby is gaining about 7oz a week and now weighs about 2lb 4oz.

Learning relaxation

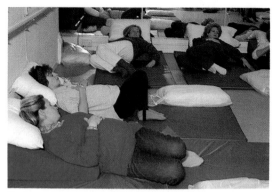

Relaxing is all about releasing the tension in your body and in your mind. Being able to relax both physically and mentally will help you during labor to counteract the natural response to pain, which is to tense your muscles and hold your breath. Imagine how you react to a stressful situation, such as a traffic jam, with shoulders hunched, teeth gritted and hands clenched. Once you can relax both during and between contractions, you will be able to work *with* them. Learning to release tension also involves correct breathing (see Week 34). If you find it difficult to relax, practice the exercises below every day.

Prenatal classes

Prenatal classes are designed to help you keep fit during your pregnancy and to prepare both you and your partner for the birth. In some really thorough classes, you'll learn basic aspects of looking after a baby. The weekly classes usually start eight to ten weeks before your baby is due.

If you're having your baby in a hospital, the hospital will probably offer classes. If you're giving birth at an out-of-hospital birth center, the center itself will probably conduct its own classes for couples planning to have their babies there. For home birth and classes emphasizing specific techniques, such as Lamaze, check the organizations listed under "Prenatal Care and Birth" (see Useful Addresses, p. 92). As a general source for classes and services in your area, the International Childbirth Education Association is probably best (see Useful Addresses, p. 92). If you're planning on having your baby in a hospital and it's nearby, it may be a good idea to go to its classes so that you can become familiar with it and its policies.

See Week 34 for Breathing for Labor

Physical relaxation

Start by getting comfortable. Either sit or lie but arrange pillows around you so that every part of your body is supported. Begin with your toes. First tense up all of the muscles in your toes and then relax them, letting them go so that they are all floppy. Then tense your feet – and let go.

Continue on up your body: your calves, thighs, buttocks, stomach and so on, right up to your face, tensing and then relaxing every single part. This should take about five minutes. Then do it again, this time beginning from the top. Continue until your whole body is as floppy as a rag doll.

Mental relaxation

Get comfortable and clear your mind of anything that's making you nervous. Then concentrate on your breathing: breathe in deeply, hold your breath for a count of five seconds, and then breathe out slowly. As you do so, make sure all your muscles are relaxed – drop your shoulders and jaw, and unclench your hands – and continue to breathe deeply.

Then let your imagination flow. Picture yourself on a beach in the sun under a blue sky, hearing the gentle noise of the waves beside you, or imagine you are floating up to the clouds. Choose whatever image appeals to you.

Relaxing with your partner

Your partner can help you to relax. He must firmly massage the part of your body that is tense so that his hands draw the tension out of you. If you have a headache, for example, let your partner stand behind you and, with two fingers, firmly press each side of your head, against your temples. As he gradually lessens the pressure, your tension will ease away. He can do the same with your shoulders, only this time using the whole of his hands rather than just his fingers. The regular rhythm of gentle stroking will help you to relax generally; this can be useful in the early stages of labor.

Week 30

Month: may Dates: 10

MON

TUES

WED

THURS

★ FRI

SAT

SUN

Notes

YOU AND YOUR DEVELOPING BABY

You During the next ten weeks your baby will be gaining about 7oz a week and you will be gaining almost twice as much. From now on you will become much larger, slower and clumsier. You may feel as if your internal organs are being squeezed out and put under pressure from your enlarging uterus.

Baby Your baby is probably lying in a curled-up position with his knees bent, his arms and legs crossed and his chin resting on his chest. He now begins to move less and to settle, and within the next two weeks will have turned upside down if he has not already done so. Most babies adopt a head down-wards position so that they can be born head first. If your baby is one of the four per cent who has his bottom downwards ('breech'' presentation) your doctor will probably try and turn him round later on.

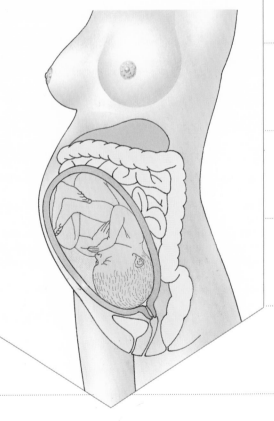

DON'T FORGET If you haven't already done so, stop smoking now. Your baby needs oxygen to enable him to grow and smoking reduces the amount he will get.

Thinking about feeding

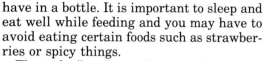

If this is your first baby you may find it hard to know how you will want to feed him. You don't have to decide now, but if you are at all uncertain it is best to start with breast-feeding, as you can always change to bottle-feeding later. It is much more difficult to breast-feed when you have started with bottle-feeding.

Breast-feeding

Breast-feeding is certainly best for the health of your baby. Breast milk contains all the nourishment he needs. It is the right temperature and right consistency and, being easily digested, is less likely to cause diarrhea, constipation or stomach upsets. Breast milk provides antibodies which help to protect your baby against coughs, colds and chest infections; it also helps prevent allergies, such as eczema and asthma.

Breast-feeding is easier and cheaper than bottle-feeding. It is also convenient – your milk is always available, even when traveling. Breast-fed babies are unlikely to get fat. They take as much milk as they need.

Breast-feeding can be emotionally satisfying for the mother. It may also help you regain your figure, due partly to the calories burned up and also because the hormones involved in breast-feeding cause "afterpains" which help your uterus to contract back to its pre-pregnancy size and position.

Some mothers find that breast-feeding can be uncomfortable or even painful at first, but this soon disappears. If you feel that breast-feeding could tie you down, remember that you can express your milk for your baby to have in a bottle. It is important to sleep and eat well while feeding and you may have to avoid eating certain foods such as strawberries or spicy things.

The only "equipment" you will need for breast-feeding are three nursing bras (you may want to wear them at night too). They should be adjustable (the size of your breasts will change) and easy to open at the front with one hand. You will also need disposable breast pads to soak up leaking milk, or you could use muslin squares.

Bottle-feeding

If you do decide to bottle-feed, there is no need to feel guilty. The most important thing in feeding is to be relaxed and hold your baby close. Some women feel that bottle-feeding will leave them freer to carry on their own life and of course it is an experience that can be shared by the father. With bottle-feeding you can see exactly how much milk your baby has taken, and some mothers find this reassuring.

You may, however, find all the sterilizing and preparation required for bottle-feeding hard work, and very time-consuming, at first. There is also a danger of your baby becoming overweight, since it is easy to overfeed with bottle formulas.

Bottle-feeding is more expensive than breast-feeding. Besides buying the powdered formula milk, you also need a lot of equipment (see below). In addition to the six bottles and nipples, you should have some form of sterilizing unit unless you are using plastic-frame nursers with disposable bags.

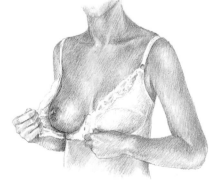

◁ *Nursing bras should be front-opening and adjustable; they should also give your breasts some support.*

In the interests of your baby's health, all bottle-feeding equipment must be sterilized before use. The powdered formula milk has to be measured and made up accurately. ▷

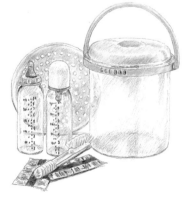

Week 31

Month:
May
MON

Dates: 17   96

TUES
May   06   03

WED

THURS

* **FRI**

SAT

SUN

Notes

You You are probably beginning to feel breathless when you overdo things, which may make you become impatient for the birth. Or, you may find yourself becoming completely absorbed with your body and your baby's movements. It can be quite a dilemma. Just take care if you do find yourself withdrawing from the world around you. Make sure you don't let your partner feel left out.

If your breasts are becoming heavy, begin wearing a well-fitting bra at night as well as during the day from now on. Good support will make them feel more comfortable.

Baby As your baby grows plumper, his skin fills out and becomes smoother. Both the vernix and the lanugo begin to disappear.

Around this week the air sacs in his lungs become lined with a layer of cells which produce a liquid called surfactant. This will prevent the air sacs from collapsing when your baby begins to breathe after birth.

This week your baby measures around 1ft 3½in and weighs about 3lb 2oz.

■ **DON'T FORGET** Never stand up when you can sit, and never sit when you can lie down.

Good posture

Backache can occur at any time during pregnancy, though the greatest risk is now. If your stomach muscles are not strong enough to carry your extra weight, your back muscles are forced to work to support your spine. This puts strain on them. It will help to learn, or relearn, how to stand, sit and lie properly.

When standing

Always stand as straight as possible and don't lean backwards. Improve your posture by wearing low (or flat) heels, tucking your buttocks in, keeping your shoulders dropped and carrying yourself as if you want the top of your head to touch the ceiling. Avoid stooping; instead kneel, sit or squat to do the ironing, peel potatoes, clean the bath etc.

When sitting

Sit well back in a chair and support your back by putting a rolled-up towel or small cushion in the hollow of your spine. Try sitting cross-legged when you can.

When lying down

Use a firm mattress and lie flat on your back or on your side. Support your body with pillows wherever they are needed – if lying on your side, try placing them under your head and upper arm; under your stomach; under your top knee and under your hips. To ease upper backache, lie flat on your back with pillows under your head and knees (provided you are comfortable lying on your back).

To get up

To avoid straining your back and abdominal muscles, roll on to your side first and push yourself up using your arm muscles.

Lifting and carrying

Avoid lifting anything heavy if you can. If you have to pick something up, squat down keeping your back straight.

If you need to carry heavy items, keep them close to your body. Distribute the weight evenly: put shopping in two bags of equal weight rather than a single heavy one.

Low backache

To relieve your spine of your baby's weight, get on all fours as often as possible. Do the cat exercise (see Week 22) whenever you can and, if you feel like it, scrub the kitchen floor daily!

See Week 24 for Discomfort in Bed

Remember to keep your back straight whenever you sit cross-legged. ▷

Squat down using your leg muscles to pick things up – it prevents straining your back. ▷

◁ Get up from a lying position by first rolling on to your side then pushing yourself up on to your elbow.

Week 32

Month: _may_   Dates: _23_

MON

TUES

WED

⋆THURS _may 15. 03_

FRI

SAT

SUN

Notes

You As your uterus rises and your baby and uterus push up under your diaphragm, the bottom edge of your ribcage may become quite sore. You may experience a loss of libido (sexual desire) during the next few weeks; on the other hand, many women find sex exciting around this time of pregnancy.

Baby Your child is now perfectly formed, although still relatively thin, and his proportions are much as you would expect them to be at birth. If he were born now he would have a very good chance of survival, because his lungs are almost developed. He would however need to be placed in an incubator as not enough insulating fat reserves have yet been deposited beneath his skin.

His movements are now very vigorous and may even be quite uncomfortable, especially if his feet get caught under your ribs; sitting up straight will help counteract this. You will probably be aware of him getting hiccups whenever he swallows some amniotic fluid. Each week he will have less and less room to move about and the "lie", the position he has taken up in the womb, will be checked to make sure he is lying head downward ready for birth. If not, your doctor will decide whether to try and turn the baby, or if special delivery techniques will be needed.

Your baby now weighs about 3lb 10oz and measures just over 1ft 4in.

DON'T FORGET Begin your prenatal classes now if you haven't already.

Getting ready

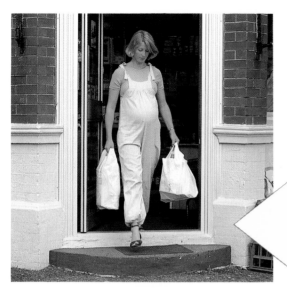

that some time in the next couple of months your life will totally change and you've got to start preparing for it now.

It's important to take things easy, especially if you are not sleeping well. Your body is going through a lot of physical stress and needs to be looked after, so rest as much as you can. But try to get out every day too. A daily walk is good exercise; it will benefit your circulation and general health. Don't go too fast or too far or the exertion may

See Weeks 27 and 28 for Shopping for Equipment

See Week 33 for Shopping for Layette

Using the time
It's worth stocking up on non-perishable items now, because you won't be able to get out for a major shopping trip for quite a while with a newborn baby.

If you haven't already finished work, you should soon be doing so, and this is the time to start planning for labor and your new family life. Your mind may be reeling with conflicting emotions: you're probably excited at the prospect of your baby being born – and yet unable to really imagine having a baby; you may be nervous about the birth itself and worried about whether your baby is going to be all right. At the same time you may even feel unsure about whether you really want a baby! The only sure thing is

make you exhausted and breathless.

On the practical level, you must get organized. Don't worry about the housework if you don't feel like doing it, but do get ready for the birth during the next few weeks. Pack your suitacse for the hospital; finish preparing your baby's room and make sure you have all the equipment and clothes you will need for him immediately. It is also a good idea to spend some time stocking your freezer, if you have one. Cook and freeze as much as you can now for the week immediately after coming out of the hospital when you won't feel like cooking, and will not have much time for it anyway.

Use this time to educate yourself too. Friends with babies will be happy to tell you what they can about looking after children. Ask their advice and get as many hints as you can. It's also useful to watch other mothers with their children and see what you think; it will help you to work out what kind of a mother you want to be with your child. Buy a book about child care to read now and to consult in the future.

On the fun side, make the most of these last days of freedom. Visit friends or have them over to lunch or dinner. Go to the theater and movies and make any frivolous shopping trips now, before you get too tired and shopping becomes a chore.

Tips for traveling
- ☐ Don't stray too far from home in the last few weeks in case labor begins.
- ☐ When traveling as a passenger in the car, you may find you have more space in the back seat.
- ☐ Stop every hour or so on a car journey and go for a short walk.
- ☐ Always take plenty to drink on a journey as you may well get thirsty.
- ☐ Remember you may need a letter from your doctor before you are allowed to travel by plane. Many airlines may not let you fly from now on, even with your doctor's permission (see Week 15).

Week 33

Month:
may

Dates:
30

MON

10/12/00

TUES

5/20/03

WED

*✳*THURS 10/12/00/33 week

FRI

SAT

SUN

Notes

You You may well find yourself becoming curious about other babies. If you have any friends who have just had a baby, visit them and watch a newborn baby's kicking movements. You may be able to match the movements to those you are feeling in your womb.

If you want to breast-feed, start giving your nipples a gentle massage daily. If you have inverted nipples and are worried about future breast-feeding problems, you could try wearing nipple shields for a few hours a day. But most problems will be solved by a hungry baby.

If you have difficulty breathing, remember to sit and stand up straight. From around Week 36 this problem should disappear as your baby's head will become 'engaged' (descend into your pelvis).

Baby By now your baby will measure about 1ft 4½in and will weigh approximately 4½lb.

Your doctor will be able to see which way up your baby is or which way he is "presenting" – see Understanding your Medical Records, page 88. He is most likely to have settled into a head downwards position, ready to be born head first. A minority of babies have their bottom downwards, known as breech position.

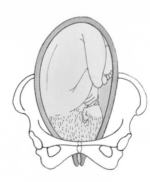 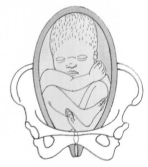

The normal position for delivery is head first.

Some babies are in a breech position, presenting bottom first.

■ **DON'T FORGET** Stand up straight at all times and rest for at least an hour a day if you can.

70

Shopping for layette

Buy just enough clothes in advance to make sure your baby can always be warm and clean over the first few weeks. Remember that babies grow quickly during the first few weeks and months, so don't buy too many of the first size(s). Bear in mind that a new baby doesn't need different clothes for day and night. The hospital may provide clothes for your baby's stay there.

Avoid buying synthetic fabrics for your baby's first weeks. They tend to increase the heat in hot weather and leave him cold when it's chilly. Avoid or remove drawstrings around the neck and make sure that any elastic is not too tight.

Baby toiletries and other items

☐ Zinc and castor oil cream, petroleum jelly or another diaper rash cream.
☐ Soft hairbrush; blunt-ended nail scissors.

☐ Baby wipes for cleaning baby's bottom, useful when you are out visiting.
☐ Pure baby soap or bath liquid.
☐ Changing bag to carry diaper equipment around in.
☐ Absorbent cotton rolls or balls.
☐ 2 soft facecloths or natural sponges and 2 soft towels: keep them for baby's use only.

Which diapers?

Disposable diapers are more convenient but are more expensive than washable ones though with washable diapers the initial outlay is high. You'll need 24–30 cloth diapers; disposable diaper liners; diaper pins; 3 pairs waterproof pants; plastic bucket and sterilizing powder or liquid.

Large economy-size packs of disposable diapers will save you money but don't stock up on too many in the small size.

See Weeks 27 and 28 for Shopping for Equipment

First baby clothes

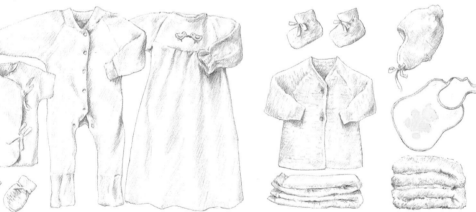

☐ 4 all-in-one stretch suits; buy them with snaps around the inside leg so that you don't have to remove the whole outfit for diaper changing. You can cut off the feet when baby has grown. Or buy nighties instead.
☐ 4 buntings or sleepsuits for daytime outings and night time sleeping in cold weather.
☐ 4 undershirts : choose cotton or thermal according to the season; an envelope neck or wrap-around style facilitates

dressing. Bodysuits which fasten between his legs don't leave a gap around the tummy.
☐ 3 cardigans/jackets: wool is most comfortable and several light layers are better than one thick one.
☐ 2 pairs mittens: for cold weather. Cotton mittens will stop a young baby scratching his face.
☐ 3 pairs booties or socks: babies' circulation is poor and

their feet get cold through not moving around. Booties are unnecessary over stretch suits and for summer babies.
☐ 2 bonnets: essential for cold weather. Babies lose most heat through their head.
☐ Sunhat: to protect a summer baby's head and eyes from the sun.
☐ 4 bibs: bibs protect his clothes in case he brings back milk.
☐ Shawl or blanket.
☐ Diapers (see above).

Week 34 96

Month: _june_

MON

TUES

WED

✱ THURS   5/28/63
28

FRI

SAT

SUN

Notes

Dates: 6

You You may now start to notice Braxton Hicks contractions beginning. They will feel like a 20–30-second hardening of your uterus and they usually occur during the last weeks of pregnancy if not before. These contractions are sometimes wrongly interpreted as signs of premature labor. Although uncomfortable, they are not painful; they are weaker and last less time than labor contractions.

Baby Your baby's skin is becoming pinker. He is beginning to be able to differentiate between light and dark and, for example, is able to see more if the sun shines on your stomach. He is also blinking.

During the first stage of labor your cervix (2), normally closed, starts to thin out and to dilate, or open. The contractions of the uterus (1) gradually draw the cervix upwards, over the baby's head.

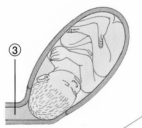

The dilatation of the cervix is measured in centimeters. At 5–6cm (2–2⅜in) you are approximately half-dilated. The baby's head is being squeezed lower in the uterus.

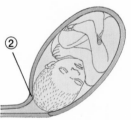

At 10cm (4in) the cervix is fully dilated. It has stretched open sufficiently to allow the baby's head to pass through the vagina (3).

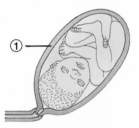

■ **DON'T FORGET** Start arranging friends, relations or paid help to come in and help you after your baby is born.

72

Breathing for labor

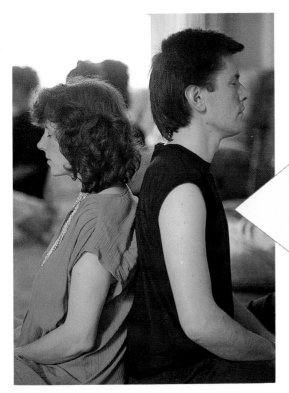

breath will always take care of itself. Do not hold your breath at any stage, as this increases tension. Breathe as deeply as is comfortable; you will find that your breathing is quite shallow when practicing at home, because you are still, but be prepared for it to get deeper in labor when you are working much harder.

Breathe in through your nose and out

See Week 29 for Learning Relaxation

See Week 37 for Onset of Labor

Breathing techniques
Breathe in through your nose and out through your mouth. Remember to breathe as smoothly as possible and as deeply as you find comfortable, concentrating on the outward breath.

Controlled breathing will help you to cope with your contractions by encouraging you to relax your muscles and by distracting your mind and body from any pain you may experience. If you go to prenatal classes you will be taught some breathing exercises and it is a good idea to practice them at home on a regular basis. During these exercises your mind should be concentrating and your body should be completely relaxed. It might help your mind to concentrate if you fix your eyes on an object in the room.

The particular exercises may vary slightly from one class to another, but the principle of breathing for labor remains the same. In some ways, the simpler the breathing the better, because if there are too many different "levels" to remember you are more likely to become muddled during the labor, which may make you feel you have lost control.

Aim to slow down your breathing, and learn to concentrate on the outward breath because this is what relaxes you. The inward

through your mouth, pursing your lips. This may seem strange when you are sitting at home, not needing to take large breaths, but will make more sense in labor when your breathing is deeper and faster. But it will take some practice.

So – take a breath in through your nose and try to make the air go down to the bottom of your lungs at the base of your ribs. If you are doing this correctly, you will find that your chest moves only a little but your abdomen is pushed out as you breathe in – put one hand on your chest and the other on your stomach to check this.

As you breathe out, relax those tense muscles – drop your shoulders and jaw and unclench your hands. If you find it difficult to release the tension that is naturally building up, stretch down your shoulders and stretch out your hands to unclench your tensed muscles. In labor, once the contraction is finished, breathe a deep sigh of relief – the pain has gone for a few minutes.

If you become breathless during your exercises, you are breathing too fast – make a conscious effort to slow down. If you become dizzy, it means that you are breathing in too strongly (hyperventilating): cup your hands tightly round your mouth and breathe normally in and out several times until you feel better. Then carry on with the exercises, making the "out" breath even stronger.

73

Week 35

Month: *June*

Dates: *13*

MON

TUES

WED

THURS

FRI

SAT

SUN

Notes

You You will need to buy three nursing bras soon, if you plan to breast-feed your baby. Have them expertly fitted as your body will be changing shape yet again. Make sure they support your breasts and that you can open (and close) each side using one hand only.

Don't stand or sit in one position for too long; not only may your ankles swell, but your body may become increasingly immobile. Rest as much of the day as you feel like.

Baby Your baby is rapidly losing his wrinkled appearance and becoming plumper. Between now and birth more fat will be deposited all over his body, mainly around the shoulders.

The hair on his head is growing and his soft toe- and fingernails have grown almost to the ends of his fingers and toes.

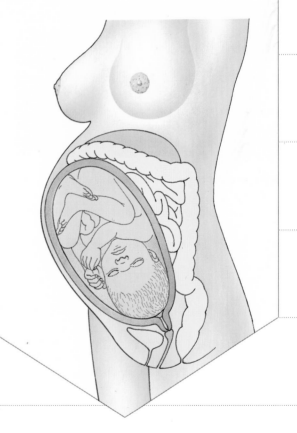

Pain relief

Labor is usually painful, to a greater or lesser degree, therefore it's a good idea to know what kinds of pain relief are readily available so you can think about, and discuss them before it all starts. However, you should always be prepared to be flexible about any decisions you make. Whatever you imagine your labor will be like, it is bound to be different in some respect.

General anesthesia

In the past, women in labor were routinely given general anesthetics but this practice is seldom used today because of complications. The use of analgesics (drugs which relieve or diminish the intensity of pain but do not cause unconsciousness) and local anesthetics (such as epidurals) is much more common. Occasionally, however, certain mild gases such as nitrous oxide, which you breathe in through a face mask that covers your mouth and nose, are used during labor. Though they do not put you to sleep, these can make it very difficult to concentrate on using other pain relief techniques, such as breathing and relaxation. They can also interfere with maternal-infant bonding and nursing immediately after delivery, but have no side-effects on your baby.

Narcotic analgesics

Narcotics, such as Demerol, are strong pain relievers which are given usually through an intravenous (i.v.) line. Most narcotic analgesics take about fifteen minutes to work and the effect lasts about two hours. Though they lessen the pain, narcotics do not entirely take it away; they may also make you drowsy. There are no serious side-effects, but narcotics can make it difficult to push and cause newborns to be slow to start breathing if they are given too near the time of delivery. Your physician will try to coordinate the narcotic dose with the estimated time of delivery. If necessary, a second drug can be given to reverse the effect if delivery turns out to be imminent.

Epidural

For most women an epidural gives complete pain relief and for a long or very painful labor it may be an ideal solution. It is a special type of local anesthetic that works by blocking the nerves which carry the feelings of pain from your uterus, cervix and vagina to your brain. It can even be used for a Cesarean section, allowing the mother to remain conscious for the birth.

The disadvantage of an epidural is that your legs and the lower half of your body are numb and you can no longer move about, or even change position, without help. Since you cannot feel your contractions you may not feel the urge to push either and will have to be told when to do so. This may mean it takes longer to push your baby out or that the baby has to be delivered by forceps.

See
Week 34 for
Breathing for
Labor

See
Week 40 for
The Birth

Having an epidural

If you know in advance that you want an epidural it is a good idea to ask as soon as you

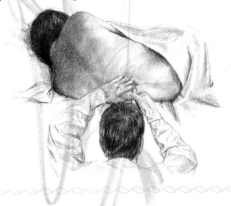

get into the labor room as the anesthetist may be in demand around the hospital.

Having an epidural is not painful, as your back is numbed before it is given. You lie curled up on your side on the edge of the bed and a needle is injected between the bones of your spine. A plastic tube is threaded down the needle into a place outside the nerves of the spinal cord. The needle is then removed and the tube is held in place on your back by some sticky tape. The anesthetic is then injected down the tube and takes about fifteen minutes to work. When it starts wearing off, between one and three hours later, further injections are given in the same way.

Week 36

Month:
Jeene

MON

Dates: 20

TUES

WED

* THURS

FRI

SAT

SUN

Notes

YOU AND YOUR DEVELOPING BABY

You The top of your uterus has reached its highest point by now – just below your breast bone. This will make breathing uncomfortable and may also give you a jabbing pain in your ribcage.

If this is your first baby, "lightening" may occur some time during the next few weeks. This is when your baby's head "engages", or drops into your pelvis, which indicates that he can pass through your pelvic cavity without difficulty. With a second or subsequent pregnancy, lightening may not occur until just before labor begins. Prenatal visits are weekly from now on.

Baby All your baby's organs are now almost mature and if he is born he has a ninety per cent chance of survival. Only his lungs may be insufficiently developed. His skin is soft and smooth and his body has fattened out.

Your baby's head has dropped into your pelvis.

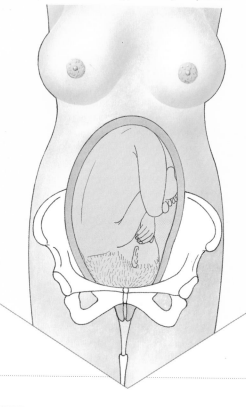

DON'T FORGET Pack your bags now.

Packing your suitcase

You will need to pack one bag solely for the labor room, containing all the equipment you might need during labor. It should be ready several weeks before your due date. Some of the items in it will need to go to the maternity ward with you, others can be taken home by your partner. Some items, such as ice cubes, can only be packed at the last minute.

The amount of luggage you take to the maternity ward will depend on the length of your hospital stay. Bear in mind that you can always ask your partner or visiting family and friends to bring in anything you have forgotten, especially perishables like crackers and fresh fruit. Many hospitals like to keep babies in hospital clothes while they are there, so you may not need any baby clothes until the day you leave. The hospital will also provide a supply of baby toiletries, such as absorbent cotton and diaper cream.

You might think it worth also packing a bag now for your partner to bring in when it is time for you to come home. This should contain some comfortable clothes for you (bearing in mind your figure will not be back to its original shape) and the baby's clothes. The most important item of all to have ready is an approved infant car safety seat for the ride home.

See Week 33 for Shopping for Layette

See Week 38 for Fathers in Labor

Labor room bag
- ☒ Mineral water atomizer, plant spray or washcloth to cool you down.
- ☐ Vacuum flask filled with ice cubes for you to suck or to use as a cold-pack for backache during contractions.
- ☐ Warm socks (you may get cold during labor).
- ☐ Lip salve or petroleum jelly.
- ☐ Towel and toilet bag containing washcloth, toothbrush and other essential toiletries.
- ☐ Hairbrush or comb; elastic to tie back long hair.
- ☐ A mirror (if you want to watch the birth).
- ☐ Nourishing snacks (sandwiches, nuts, raisins, chocolate) to sustain your partner during a long labor.
- ☐ Glucose tablets to give you strength during the first stage.
- ☐ Radio, personal stereo or portable television if they will help you relax; find out if they are allowed in the labor room.
- ☐ Camera (if you want your partner to photograph the birth).
- ☐ A comfortable cotton nightgown (front-fastening if you plan to breast-feed).
- ☐ Nursing bra; cotton or paper underpants.
- ☐ Coins for the pay telephone.

Maternity ward suitcase
- ☐ 2 extra nightgowns.
- ☐ Slippers, bedjacket and robe.
- ☐ Address book, writing paper and pen.
- ☐ 2 packs stick-on sanitary napkins.
- ☐ Another washcloth (use one on each breast in a hot bath to relieve engorged breasts).
- ☐ Earplugs and eyeshades to help you sleep.
- ☐ Other toiletries such as shampoo, soap, deodorant, face creams and make-up.
- ☐ Tissues and/or soft toilet paper.
- ☐ A tube of lanolin cream to help with sore nipples.
- ☐ 2 extra nursing bras; breast pads.
- ☐ Rubber ring (to sit on if you have an episiotomy).
- ☐ Drinks for you and your guests, such as apple or grape juice.
- ☐ A book to help you relax.
- ☐ Cooking salt (put a handful in each bath to help heal stitches).
- ☐ Diapers. (Check with the hospital if you are expected to bring your own).

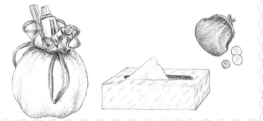

Week 37

Month: _June_

Dates: _27_

MON

TUES

WED

★ **THURS** _The First backache & a little contraction_

FRI

SAT

SUN

Notes

GET READY NOW

Although it would be most convenient if your baby was born the day he was due, this is unlikely to be the case. He could be born any day from now until the end of Week 42. The average duration of a twin pregnancy is only 37 weeks so prepare yourself now if they haven't yet appeared. Second, third and fourth babies are also more often early than late.

☐ If you have a family, finalize all arrangements for your children to be cared for while you're away.

☐ Make sure you know where your partner is at all times – ask him to leave all his telephone numbers with you.

☐ Keep your car filled with gas and put a blanket in the back for comfort on the journey to the hospital. If you plan to go by taxi, keep the telephone numbers of at least two 24-hour taxi companies by your phone.

☐ If you haven't done so, pack all your bags now.

☐ Get your baby's room, layette and crib ready. Make sure his room is clear of junk and that it can be made warm the moment he comes home.

☐ Ask at least four neighbors if you can call on them to take you to the hospital should you need to go when your partner's not around.

Important telephone numbers	
Partner at work:	Neighbors:
Doctor's office:	Your parents:
Midwife/Hospital:	Partner's parents:
	Local ambulance:
	Taxi

DON'T FORGET If you're at all worried, call the hospital: better to be safe than sorry.

Onset of labor

Even though you may not believe this now, you *will* probably know when you are in labor. There's no point having sleepless nights worrying over whether tonight is going to be the night. No one has ever had a baby in their sleep. You'll be woken up if anything is about to happen, and, if it's not, you need to get all the rest you can to keep you as fit as possible for the actual day.

The most obvious "signs" to watch out for are described below and one or more of them will indicate that labor has started. However, you may not have any such definite signs. Should you experience any of the three sensations listed below, or if you are at any time worried, call your hospital (or midwife, if you're having your baby at home or at a birthing center) and tell them. Don't worry that you might be raising a false alarm: doctors are used to this. Any doctor would prefer to check and see whether you are in labor, even if you are subsequently sent home, than have you delivered into his or her safe hands too late.

Contractions The muscles of your womb will start to tighten up and will feel rather like bad period pains or a fist clenching. This is a labor contraction and it will feel quite different (stronger and more pronounced) from the Braxton Hicks contractions that have taken place throughout your pregnancy. The contractions may be accompanied by backache, nausea, wind or diarrhea.

When these contractions come strongly and regularly, labor has definitely started. Time the spaces between your contractions and when they are coming about every ten minutes, or earlier if you can't cope any longer telephone the hospital.

With a second or subsequent baby, contractions are likely to remain quite mild and infrequent until labor is advanced. They can then suddenly change to long, strong contractions, so don't delay calling the hospital.

A "show" This is when the plug of mucus at the cervix (neck of the uterus) comes away as the uterus starts to open. You may notice a small discharge of blood-streaked jelly when you go the toilet. Telephone the hospital, tell them that you have had a "show", and they will tell you what to do.

Rupturing of the membranes This is when the bag of amniotic fluid in which your baby was floating breaks and the amniotic fluid starts to come out. It is known as "the waters breaking". This usually happens towards the end of the first stage of labor but may happen at the onset of labor or several days before. You'll notice either a small leak or a gush of warm fluid escaping from your vagina. It may feel like a period starting and it may be accompanied by some bleeding. Telephone the hospital at once.

See Week 36 for Packing Your Suitcase

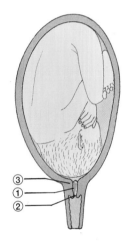

The sticky plug of mucus (1) that seals the cervical canal (2) during pregnancy is dislodged once the cervix (3) begins to dilate. The slightly blood-stained, jelly-like discharge is known as "the show" when it is released. It may not mean that labor has started, although it indicates that your cervix is opening a little. It may not be dislodged until labor is well under way.

Telephone the hospital immediately if ...
- ☐ Your waters break.
- ☐ You have any bleeding. If you are bleeding heavily, rest with your feet up until an ambulance arrives.
- ☐ Your contractions are coming every ten minutes and your waters break.
- ☑ Your contractions are coming more frequently than every ten minutes or are painful.

Remember to allow for the time it will take to get you to the hospital, so don't delay telephoning the hospital for too long. Tell your partner not to drive too fast to the hospital: a nerve-racking, bumpy ride can have a worse effect on you than simply arriving at the hospital a few minutes later.

Week 38

Month: *July*

Dates: *4*

MON

TUES

WED

* **THURS**

FRI

SAT *38/ For Elizabeth*
July /weeks 9 6
6 13oz 19 inch. 6

SUN

Notes

You You may feel bulky and a little bored with your pregnancy by now, or may be getting depressed about having your baby. Rest, carry on taking gentle exercise, have your hair cut and go to the movies in order to distract yourself. Don't be alarmed by any shooting pains in your groin and down your legs – they are perfectly normal. It probably means that your baby's head has engaged and is moving against your pelvic floor muscles or resting on a nerve. On the whole, however, he is probably moving about less.

Baby The fine lanugo hair covering your baby's body will begin to disappear, although some may remain on his shoulders and in the creases of his body.

Your baby may be trying to breathe, to practice using his lungs, and as there is no air available, he swallows amniotic fluid into his windpipe, which gives him hiccups.

Your baby may be putting on up to 1oz a day in weight, but your weight will probably remain steady from now on.

DON'T FORGET Look at these pages with your partner.

Fathers in labor

Labor is one of the hardest, most emotional and most painful experiences you will go through together. Labor itself, and the way you will feel during it, are totally unpredictable for both of you. At worst you will snap at your partner, tell him you hate him being there, scream when he touches you – and bellow at him to shut up when he asks you how he can help. At some stage you are bound to tell him you'll never have another child, and – at that moment – you will mean it! To prepare your partner for your (and his) unpredictability, ask him to read this:

Fathers, be prepared for all of this and don't hold it against your partner. Instead, support her and tell her she is being very brave. Your presence will be invaluable if you can just second-guess what she wants. Make yourself invisible when she doesn't need you.

Remember that you are on the same side. Respect your partner's wishes and allow

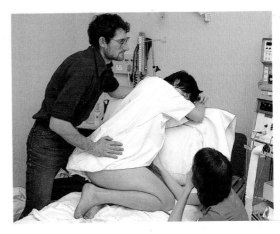

See
Week 23 for
The Father's
Role

See
Week 36 for
Packing Your
Suitcase

that she may change her mind. You're not experiencing the pain – she is. If she now wants an epidural having talked about "natural childbirth", that's fine. Give comfort in any way you can.

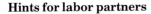

Hints for labor partners

- ☐ Your role will begin the moment your partner starts labor (make sure you know what the signs are, see Week 37). It is especially important *before* you get to the hospital, when there is no one else around. Work through her relaxation and breathing techniques now, before labor proper.
- ☐ Do not try to plan ahead too much or to anticipate events, because labor can take any shape or form. Keep an open mind and remember there is no "right" or "wrong".
- ☐ No matter how useless you may feel at some points during labor, be reassured that your very presence is supportive. Yours is a familiar face in a strange atmosphere and that will be comforting in itself. If your partner is unhappy about something, she can turn to you and you can do something about it. If she is confined to bed, you can be her legs and voice.
- ☐ During contractions you can "breathe" with her, especially if you see she's getting in a muddle and needs reinforcement. In the early stages, you can walk around with her and let her lean against you.

- ☐ Make sure she is well supported and relaxed at all times. During labor see that she has enough pillows behind her, and stroke her if it would help. She may like you to apply a gentle fingertip massage to her stomach, thighs or shoulders. But don't feel rejected if she wants to be left alone.
- ☐ Always be relaxed yourself. It may be enough for you to just sit in the corner of the room reading or doing a crossword. Ask the doctor or nurse if there's anything you could be doing to help.
- ☐ During labor if your partner says she is in pain, agree with her. Don't pretend the pain isn't there – you are downgrading her experience. Instead, congratulate her on how well she is doing.
- ☐ If you are asked to leave the room because the doctor or midwife wants to examine your partner in private, make sure *she* wants you to leave. If she doesn't, courteously ask if you can stay.
- ☐ Giving birth is a highly emotional state. Don't be surprised if your partner gets upset and if you, too, find yourself slightly overwhelmed and disturbed emotionally.

Week 39

Month: _july_   Dates: _11_

MON

TUES

WED

✱ THURS

FRI NOU 24 2:5 AM
39/weeks For Adriana
6 12oz 2/ınch.   21 1/2 Lenght

SAT

SUN

Notes

YOU AND YOUR DEVELOPING BABY

You If this is your first baby, your womb will now be approximately three fingers below your breast bone – as in Week 32 – if lightening has occurred.

You will probably be feeling quite exhausted by now and may just want to stay at home with your feet up. Do just that – rest is essential. If, however, your "nesting instinct" makes you want to rush around organizing and tidying everything up, that's all right too – but don't take on too much and don't strain or stretch your body.

Baby Your baby's intestine is filled with meconium, a sticky, dark greenish-black substance made up of the excretions from his alimentary glands mixed with bile pigment, lanugo and cells from the bowel wall. This will be his first bowel movement, which will be passed during the first two days of his life, and possibly also during labor, so don't be shocked when you see it.

DON'T FORGET For an active birth you need a support partner or two.

Positions during labor

There are as many different labor positions as there are women, so it's important to get your body into some of them now to see which feel comfortable. At the time you will rely more on instinct to choose the right one. No matter which birthing position you choose, it is important to give your baby as much room as possible. This can be achieved by holding your knees well apart and allowing your uterus to tilt forward on to your abdominal wall, away from your spine.

Some hospitals prefer women in labor to be lying down, though many now have a more open-minded attitude. You may feel you want a more active labor, during which you stand, sit, kneel, rock, walk about or squat. Bear in mind that an active birth means you need a support partner (or two). It also means you can't have an epidural.

If you want an active birth it is important that you discuss your views with your doctor well in advance (see Week 9); you may have to find a hospital that has the facilities for women to be active during labor, such as adjustable beds for birth.

It is imperative that you trust the medical staff who are delivering your baby and co-operate with them. Don't be upset if you end up lying on a hospital bed unable to move, with a fetal monitor strapped around your belly or an intravenous drip in your arm. The richness of your labor experience won't be lessened, it will just be different.

See Week 31 for Good Posture

See Week 9 for Prenatal Care

Active Birth? Pros and Cons

- [ ] If you are left to find the position that suits you, your pain may be reduced.
- [ ] Squatting or kneeling puts your pelvis and pelvic organs in the best position to deliver your baby.
- [ ] If you are upright you have the force of gravity on your side.
- [ ] In an upright position your uterus won't press on the large veins leading to the heart, which may give your baby a better chance of getting his oxygen supply.
- [ ] Being upright can promote stronger contractions in the first stage. This may lessen the need for forceps or episiotomy.
- [ ] An upright position allows for spontaneous delivery of the placenta.
- [ ] Lying down may be more restful for you.
- [ ] If you're lying down it's easier for the doctor and midwife to examine you.

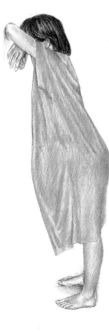

The most conventional birthing position in hospital is lying on your back with several pillows under your head, pulling your thighs towards you and pushing your feet against two stirrups. ▷

Going down on all fours, like a dog, relieves low backache and reduces pressure on the umbilical cord. This position also helps if your baby's broad shoulders get stuck. ▽

◁ *If contractions are weakening, stand facing a wall with your feet well apart and lean forward, placing your lower arms under your head on the wall. This lets your uterus become as spherical as possible.*

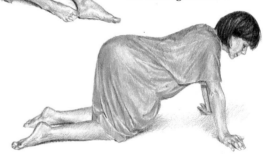

Week 40

Month: _july_

MON

Dates: 18

TUES

WED

*THURS

FRI

SAT

SUN

Notes

You You may be getting quite nervous as the expected date of delivery approaches. After all, pregnancy is now quite a familiar state! Only five per cent of babies arrive on their due date, but you may well be one of the lucky ones.

Baby His skin is soft and smooth and most of the lanugo has disappeared. His body is completely covered with vernix.

Don't get a shock when you see him for the first time. He may be blue in color, some of his head and body will still be covered with white, cheesy-looking vernix, and may also be smeared with your blood. He will be wet and slippery, his hair will have stuck to his face and he will probably be pulling an angry face just before taking his first breath; in addition, his head may still have a strange shape after the passage down the birth canal. Never mind – he's there and he's safe. You won't be looking that great either!

Your fully developed baby is soon to leave your womb.

DON'T FORGET Give up all preconceptions, and keep a flexible attitude of mind throughout the birth.

The birth

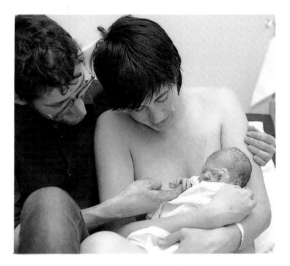

There is no such thing as the perfect birth. Nor is there such a thing as failure in labor, as there is no standard to be achieved. Each labor is highly individual and you should be prepared to work with whatever your own labor brings.

You will have lived through your baby's birth countless times in your mind, but this time it will be for real. It is unlikely to be as you have imagined and, realistically, it may well be worse. Remember that whatever pain you are going through *will* end. There are drugs to help you through it, should you want them. On the day everyone will be on your side, so let them help you. But remember that labor is something *you* are doing.

Tell the hospital staff what kind of labor you are hoping for and listen to their advice as to how to achieve it. Don't be disappointed if you can't have the "natural" birth you planned for. All births are natural and there is certainly nothing artificial about your baby. Equally, don't geel bad if the "bonding" with your baby isn't immediate; it may take time to get to know each other.

The first stage

The first stage is when your cervix, which is usually closed, starts to dilate or open up. Your contractions, caused by the muscles of the womb shrinking, will slowly open up your cervix until it is about 10cm (4in) wide and ready to let your baby through.

Concentrate on the relaxation and breathing you learned to do. Take each contraction at a time and don't let anyone or anything interfere with them. Don't feel you need to be polite during a contraction; no one expects you to. In fact shouting or swearing is a good way of releasing tension!

Your contractions will gradually get stronger and more painful and you may start feeling you want to push (this is known as the "transition" stage). To stop yourself pushing, lift your head and blow out in little puffs of air, or pant, with your mouth, legs and pelvic floor completely relaxed.

You will probably be moving about for most of the first stage. If you have backache, try sitting astride a chair or kneel on all fours.

The second stage

The second stage of labor is when your baby is born. Your cervix should be fully dilated before you start pushing. Keep your chin tucked well down and your mouth closed as you give long, slow pushes. Rest between contractions, to conserve all your energy and strength for the next push.

The third stage

The third stage is the delivery of the placenta. This stage is usually very quick and easy. As your baby is born, you'll probably be given an injection in your thigh to help your womb contract. A final contraction will then push out the placenta. Any necessary stitching up will be done next. This is your first opportunity to see and hold your baby.

Induction

There are many reasons why your labor might have to be started artificially. It could be that you have high blood pressure or diabetes, or your baby is some weeks late.

The most popular method of induction is known as ARM (artificial rupture of the membranes). Your membranes are pierced, allowing some of the amniotic fluid to escape. By altering the pressure in your womb this causes labor to start. Another method is by dripping a synthetic hormone directly into your bloodstream.

See Week 35 for Pain Relief

See Week 37 for Onset of Labor

See page 86 for The Maternity Ward

See Week 34 for Dilatation of the Cervix

The maternity ward

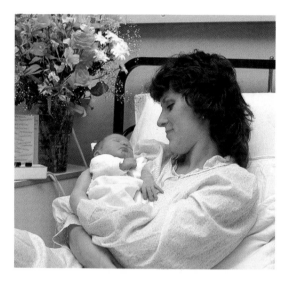

Life on the maternity ward may seem like coming down to earth with a bump after the experience you have just been through, but you have a period of great adjustment ahead and should make the most of these few days in the hospital. Use the time to get to know your baby, to learn how to care for him with the help and expertise of the hospital staff. Spend some time looking after yourself too.

The hospital environment may be an unfamiliar one, but this will be the only time you can concentrate exclusively on you and your baby without domestic responsibilities.

Getting to know your baby
In many hospitals today you can request to have your baby in a crib by your side most of the time so that you have ample opportunity to get to know each other. Don't worry if you don't feel an immediate "bond" with your baby – some mothers simply take longer than others to establish that close relationship.

It may come as a bit of a shock that you are expected to look after your baby single-handedly from day one. You are bound to feel unsure about how to handle him and what to do when he cries. But take it gently – trust your instincts and give him lots of cuddles. The hospital staff are there to help and will show you how to change a diaper

and how to bath your baby. Don't hesitate to ask them for advice about anything else which may be worrying you. By the time you leave the hospital, you will probably have covered many aspects of your baby's everyday care and you should be feeling a lot more confident.

The hospital routine
Most maternity wards have a fairly strict routine and you will be expected to fit into it. You may find elements of this difficult, such as the early start to the day, and regulated visiting hours but the routine is designed for the ward to run smoothly. The doctors usually do their rounds in the morning and will check on you and the baby; the afternoons are generally more restful and there is usually a period of enforced quiet – use it!

Life on the maternity ward may at times seem like being back at school, with communal bathrooms and the general background hubbub. Use the opportunity to discuss your experiences or any anxieties with other new mothers.

Although you may want to share the excitement of your baby with all your friends and family, bear in mind that visitors can be very tiring, especially in the first few days. It is also important to spend some time alone with your partner.

Looking after yourself
Use the time in the hospital to get yourself in good condition for your return home. Get as much rest as you can and start your postnatal exercises (see below).

If you have had an exhausting labor, you can ask the hospital staff to look after your baby for the first night so that you can catch up on lost sleep. Nobody will think the worse of you for this; you can always ask to be woken if he needs feeding. On the other hand your emotional "high" may stop you from sleeping during the first night after delivery – you may still be too excited, or may find yourself re-living the birth every time you close your eyes.

The physical strain of labor may make you ache severely and it may be a great effort to drag yourself to the bathroom for the first day or so. If you had an episiotomy, your stitches may give you pain, or at least discomfort, especially when you sit down; sitting on a rubber ring or an ice pack will help to relieve the pressure. Warm baths and using salt in the bath water will help to heal the stitched area. If you are suffering a lot of discomfort, don't be afraid to ask for painkillers or sleeping pills: they will help you to get through the first day or two, after which you will begin to feel stronger and more comfortable anyway.

You may suffer from constipation for a few days after the birth. This can be aggravated if you are worried about your stitches bursting (which they will not). Drink plenty of liquid, and eat fresh fruit and vegetables and "roughage" cereals, to ensure that the first bowel movement is soft enough to pass without too much difficulty. If necessary the doctor will suggest some medication.

You will find you bleed quite heavily for a few days after the birth and that you continue to have a brown discharge for several weeks after that. Use sanitary napkins and not internal tampons.

Breast-feeding

It can take a few days to get breast-feeding under control, and it may be painful at first, but don't be afraid to ask for help from the nurses or midwives on the ward. Your breasts will feel tender and become "engorged", or rock hard, around the third or fourth day when the milk first comes in. Your nipples may also become sore when your baby first begins to suck. But persevere – all these initial problems will be overcome.

Postnatal blues

You may well feel a bit depressed a few days after your baby is born. The level of hormones present in your bloodstream during pregnancy quickly decreases after the birth and your body has to adjust accordingly.

Whatever happens during your time on the maternity ward, don't worry or be discouraged when things go wrong. Remind yourself what an emotional and tiring experience you've been through. The next wonder of nature is that in a few months you'll have forgotten almost all of it, as you settle into your new life as a mother. You'll have just one beautiful souvenir – your baby.

Postnatal exercises

Exercise is very important after giving birth. You can start Kegal exercises, for toning the muscles of your pelvic floor, as soon as you feel able.

Strenuous exercises should not be done for at least six weeks after delivery. These include lying on your back and either lifting both legs up and then lowering them, or 'bicycling' with both legs raised.

Most of the exercises can be done in bed or, later on, lying on the floor. Do each one six times, relaxing after each. Continue them for at least six weeks after the birth.

Days 1 and 2 after birth

1. Lie on your back with your legs straight and slightly apart. Bend and stretch your ankles, then your toes, then circle your feet in both directions.

2. Lie on your back with your knees bent and your feet resting on the bed or floor. Tighten your buttock muscles and pull in your abdomen so that your back is pressed against the bed. Hold for six, then relax.

Day 3 after the birth

Introduce the following to the above exercises:

3. Practice your pelvic floor exercise (see Week 17) lying on your bed with knees bent.

Day 4 after the birth

Introduce the following:

4. Lie with your right knee bent and your right foot on the bed and your left leg straight. Slide the heel of your left leg up and down the bed, keeping the leg straight and using only your waist muscles. Change legs.

5. Lie with your knees bent and your feet on the bed. Pull in your abdominal muscles and reach across your body to place one hand on the opposite side of the bed at hip level. Return that hand to its starting position and do the same with the other hand.

Understanding your medical records

At some point you may want to take a look at your medical records. Because doctors and hospitals are often reluctant to provide access to medical records, you may be asked to put your request in writing first or go in person to the hospital's medical records department. Call the health care provider whose records you wish to see and ask what procedure you should follow.

Most of the abbreviations that you will see on your prenatal record are explained below. If there is anything that you do not understand, or if you simply can't read the doctor's writing, ask for it to be explained.

Date
The date of your prenatal visit.

Weeks
The length of your pregnancy in weeks, from the first day of your last menstrual period.

Uterine size/Height of fundus
This is the distance in centimeters from your pelvis to the top of your womb, i.e. the length of your fundus (see Week 20). The figure should be roughly the same as that in the "Weeks" column.

Urine Alb. Sugar
This shows the result of your urine tests for protein and sugar. "Tr" or "+" means a trace (or quantity) has been found. "Alb" stands for albumin, one of the proteins that could be found in your urine. "Ketones" means you are low in energy. "NAD", "Nil", or a tick all mean nothing abnormal discovered.

B.P.
Blood Pressure. This should stay at about the same level throughout pregnancy. If it goes up it can be dangerous for your baby.

Weight
This is your weight in pounds (see Week 25).

Presentation and position
This shows which way up your baby is lying or "presenting". "Vx" means vertex; "C" or "ceph" means cephalic. Both words literally mean the top of the head and show that your baby has settled into a head downwards position and is ready to be born head first. "Breech" means that your baby has his bottom downwards. "ECV" (external cephalic version) shows that your baby has been turned round by a doctor pressing on your abdomen so that your baby now has his head downwards for birth. "PP" means presenting part – the bit of your baby that is coming first.

Up to about week 30 your baby moves about a lot and then usually settles down.

Relation of PP to Brim
This is where your baby's head (the "presenting part") is situated in relation to the brim of your pelvis. "E" or "Eng" means engaged. That is when your baby's head has dropped into your pelvis ready for birth. This may not happen until a few weeks

LAB TESTS		DATE		RESULTS	
A.B.O. BLOOD GROUP					
Rhesus Blood Group					
Antibodies					
VDRL					
RUBELLA ANTIBODIES					
HEPATITIS SCREEN					
Cx SMEAR					

DATE	WEEKS	UTERINE SIZE	URINE ALB. SUGAR	B.P.	WEIGHT
3.20.89	13+6		NAD	110/60	176
4.24.89	18+	18	NAD	110/70	179
5.21.89	22	22	NAD	110/60	181.5
6.18.89	26	26	NAD	110/60	182.5
6.29.89	28		NAD	110/60	187
7.3.89	30		NAD	110/60	191
8.3.89	33+		NAD	110/60	200
9.4.89	37+	37	trace protein	110/70	201
9.18.89	39+5		NAD	105/70	207

before his birth or not until you are in labor. The engaging of your baby's head is expressed in fifths. So 1/5th means he is beginning to engage, 2/5ths means he has dropped further down and so on. "NE" means not engaged.

Abbreviations are also used to describe the way your baby is lying in your abdomen. The "O" stands for occiput (the crown of your baby's head); the "R" and "L" for whether the baby is on the right or left side of your body and the "A" and "P" for whether your baby's back is facing to the front (anterior) or to the back (posterior) of your body. So "ROA" means your baby is on the right side of your body, his back facing the front.

FH

"FHH", or "H", or a tick means fetal heart heard. "FHNH" is fetal heart not heard. "FMF" is fetal movements felt.

Edema

This is the swelling, usually of your hands, feet and ankles (see Week 24) which can lead to further problems. "+" means you have edema and each further "+" denotes the degree of swelling.

Hb

"Hb" stands for hemoglobin. This is tested in your blood to see whether you are anemic. "Fe" means that iron has been prescribed.

Next visit

The approximate date of the next visit to your doctor or midwife is written in this column. 4/52 means four weeks' time, 1/52 means in one week's time and so on.

Sig.

This is where your doctor or midwife puts his initials after giving you your checkup.

PRENATAL RECORD

DRUGS	FIRST EXAMINATION	∝ FETOPROTEIN	FIRST ULTRASOUND EXAMN.	SPECIAL POINTS TO WATCH
	Height	SERUM:—	Date: 4/24/89	
	Breasts	Date		
	Heart	OTHER TESTS	Maturity 18+/40	
ALLERGIES	Lungs			
	Varicose Veins		Placental Site: ↗ posterior	
	Pelvis			
			Other Findings FH ✓	

PRESENTA-TION AND POSITION	RELATION OF P.P. TO BRIM	F.H.	EDEMA	Hb	NEXT VISIT	SIG.	COMMENTS & RESULTS OF PRENATAL EXAMINATIONS
		NIL	88		4/52	PCB	
—	—	Scan	NIL	10.9 iron	4/52	CGN	AFP taken
✓	—	✓	NIL		4/52	AR	
					4/52	AR	
					4/52	CGN	
VX					4/52	PCB	
					4/52	KM	
Ceph	ROA	FHH	+	10.3	2/52	KM	Head Engaging
Ceph	4/5	++			1/52	PCB	

	PLANNED DISCHARGE	POSTNATAL EXAMINATION AND FAMILY PLANNING VISIT
	@ 48 HOURS	BY:
	@ 5 DAYS	HOSPITAL CLINIC
	@ 9 DAYS	
	@ OTHER	GP

Glossary

Afterbirth
See Placenta

Amniocentesis
A test sometimes performed during pregnancy which is used to detect chromosomal disorders such as Down's syndrome. It is usually done only if it is thought there may be a risk of your child suffering from one of these disorders (see Week 17).

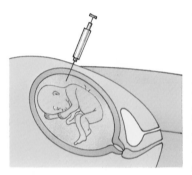

Amniotic sac
Inside your uterus your baby is floating in an oval bag formed of two thin tissues (membranes) called the amniotic sac. It is filled with waters (amniotic fluid) which cushion the baby from any knocks and jolts during pregnancy. Before or during labor, the membranes will break and the amniotic fluid will leak out. This is called 'breaking the waters' (see Week 37).

Analgesia
An analgesic is a pain-easing agent which does not cause unconsciousness. The analgesic that is most commonly used in labor is Meperidine (trade name Demerol). But your doctor may prefer another. (see Week 35).

Braxton Hicks contractions
These are thought to be the uterus's way of preparing for the contractions of labor (see Contractions). They occur every twenty minutes throughout pregnancy, although you may only notice them during the last few weeks. They feel like a painless but uncomfortable hardening across the stomach (see Week 23).

Breech presentation
Most babies are born head first, that is, the head is the presenting part. A baby in a breech presentation means that his bottom is presenting and he will come out bottom (or, in rare cases, legs) first. Only about three in every hundred babies are breech. If your baby is in a breech presentation your doctor will try and turn him round before birth.

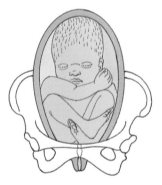

Cervix
This is the neck of your uterus, the bit which looks like the narrow part of the pear (see Uterus). It is 1in (2.5cm) long and when you are not pregnant remains almost completely closed with just a small opening through which blood passes during your monthly period. During labor muscular contractions gradually open up the cervix more and more until it is about 10cm (4in) wide, so that your baby can pass through it, and into your vagina.

Contractions
Regular tightening of the muscles of the uterus. During labor these become more forceful and will push your baby down the birth canal (see also Braxton Hicks contractions).

EDC/Due date
Expected date of confinement or expected date of delivery.

Embryo
The embryo is your baby in the early stages of pregnancy. As it grows more like a baby it becomes known as a "fetus", usually from Week 7.

Engaged
About Week 36 in a first pregnancy (later for second and subsequent pregnancies), your baby's head will drop down (engage) into your pelvis so the widest part of his head is

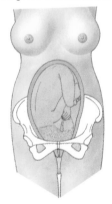

through your pelvic brim. This will make labor easier and will also help you to breathe. Another term for this is "lightening".

Most babies are born head first and will have engaged in your pelvis before labor begins.

Epidural
An anesthetic used in labor to relieve your pain while leaving you fully conscious. It is done by an injection into the fluid surrounding your spinal cord (see Week 35).

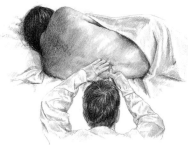

Episiotomy
An incision made in your perineum just before your baby is born in order to enlarge the exit for him and to prevent you tearing.

Fallopian tubes
Two narrow tubes about 4in long which lead from your ovaries to your uterus.

Fetus
See Embryo

Fundus
The top of your uterus (see Week 20).

Gestation
The period from conception to birth (i.e. nine months).

Hormones
Chemicals produced by the body to perform functions in particular to do with growth and reproduction. They have a variety of effects during pregnancy.

Induction
Any process which starts labor artificially (see Week 40).

Labor
The process of childbirth.

Lanugo
A growth of fine hair which will appear all over your baby's body during pregnancy (see Week 16).

Lightening
See Engaged

Membranes
See Amniotic sac

Miscarriage
The loss of a baby before twenty-eight weeks' gestation. The risk of miscarriage is highest in the first twelve weeks of pregnancy.

Mucus
See Plug of mucus

Ovaries
There are two ovaries (female sex glands) in your body, each of which is about the size of a large almond. Every month one of them expels an egg, or ovum, which weaves its way down the Fallopian tube in search of male sperm on the way up from the vagina.

Perineum
The area between your vagina and anus.

Placenta
An organ grown solely to nourish your baby and to excrete his waste products. It is a more or less circular piece of tissue, attached on the one side to your uterus and on the other to your baby via his umbilical cord. The placenta works like a sieve, allowing oxygen, food and protective antibodies to be passed from you to your baby, but in the same way toxic substances (see Week 2) can be filtered through as well. The placenta also passes your baby's waste products to you for disposal. The placenta, or "afterbirth", is expelled through the vagina shortly after your baby is born in what is known as the third stage of labor.

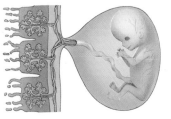

Plug of mucus
Placed in the cervix, like a cork in the neck of a bottle, the plug of mucus seals off the contents of your uterus from outside

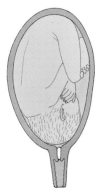

interference and protects your baby from infection. The plug comes out in order for the waters to break (see Week 37). (See also Amniotic sac)

Primagravida

A woman pregnant for the first time. An "elderly primagravida", in medical terms, is anyone having a first baby over the age of twenty-five.

Quickening

The first movements of your baby inside the uterus.

Rubella

Another name for German measles (see Week 2).

Scan

See Ultrasound scan

Stillbirth

The delivery of a baby who has already died in the uterus after twenty-eight weeks of pregnancy.

Trimester

Pregnancy is divided into three trimesters (literally thirds of pregnancy). The first is the first thirteen weeks of pregnancy, the second lasts from Week 14 to Week 27 and the third is from Week 28 until delivery (see Week 4).

Ultrasound scan

A highly sophisticated instrument which uses sound-waves to show the development of the baby in your uterus (see Week 16).

Umbilical cord

This is the link between you (your placenta) and your baby. Blood circulates through the cord, carrying oxygen and food to your baby and removing waste. The cord measures about 2ft. (See also Placenta)

Uterus

Before impregnation your uterus (womb) is about the same shape and size as a small, upside-down pear, weighs about 2oz and is hollow with a thick muscular wall. At the top it is joined on either side to the Fallopian tubes; the other, narrow end is called the cervix.

When you become pregnant the fertilized egg imbeds itself in the lining of the uterus and your unborn baby remains in there until the end of your pregnancy. By the time your baby is fully formed, the uterus is a powerful 2lb muscle-mass capable of pushing your baby out.

Vagina

Your vagina is a tube of muscle about 3–4in long which leads from your cervix to your vulva, your external sexual organs. The vagina forms the birth canal during labor.

Womb

See Uterus

When writing for information please enclose a stamped addressed envelope.

PRENATAL CARE AND BIRTH
National Center for Education in Maternal and Child Health
38 and R Streets, N.W.
Washington D.C. 20057
202-625-8400

American Academy of Husband-Coached Childbirth
P.O. Box 5224
Sherman Oaks, CA 91413
818-788-6662
800-423-2397 (toll-free outside CA)
800-42-BIRTH (toll-free CA only)
Information and referrals to prenatal classes emphasizing the Bradley/Dick-Read method

American Society of Psychoprophylaxis in Obstetrics
1840 Wilson Blvd., Suite 204
Arlington, VA 22201
703-525-7802
800-368-4404 (toll-free)
Information and referrals to prenatal classes emphasizing Lamaze techniques

International Childbirth Education Association
P.O. Box 20048
Minneapolis, MN 55420
612-854-8660
Information regarding all types of maternity services in your area

Maternity Center Association
48 E. 92nd St.
New York, NY 10128
212-369-7300
Information regarding informed childbirth and especially "natural childbirth"

Cesarean Prevention Movement
P.O. Box 152
Syracuse, NY 13210
315-424-1942
Information and referrals

American College of Nurse-Midwives
1522 K St. N.W.
Suite 1120
Washington, D.C. 20005
202-347-5445
Registry of nurse/midwives throughout U.S.

Useful addresses

National Association of Childbearing Centers
Box 1, Route 1
Perkiomenville, PA 18074
215-234-8068
Send $1 donation for list of out-of-hospital birth centers

SHARE
c/o St. Elizabeth's Hospital
211 S. Third St.
Belleville, IL 62222
618-234-2415
Support for parents who have lost a newborn through miscarriage, stillbirth, ectopic pregnancy or early infant death

POSTNATAL SUPPORT
LaLeche League International
9616 Minneapolis Ave.
Franklin Park, IL 60131
312-455-7730
Breastfeeding information and support (check phone directory for local chapter or write to above address)

March of Dimes Birth Defects Foundation
1275 Mamaroneck Ave.
White Plains, NY 10605
914-428-7100
800-626-2410 (toll-free)
Provides many publications and resources on birth defects; organizes support groups

Parents of Prematures
P.O. Box 3046
Kirkland, WA 98083
206-283-7466
Support and information for parents who have experienced the birth and hospitalization of a premature or sick baby

Parents Without Partners
8807 Colesville Road
Silver Spring, MD 20910
301-588-9354
800-637-7974 (toll-free)
Mutual support groups for single parents and their children

Parent Care
101½ S. Union St.
Alexandria, VA 22314
703-836-4678
Information and support for parents of premature and high-risk infants

National Organization of Mothers of Twins Clubs Inc.
12404 Princess Jeanne N.E.
Albuquerque, NM 87112-4640
505-275-0955

National Down Syndrome Congress
1800 Dempster St.
Park Ridge, IL 60068-1146
312-823-7550 (IL only)
800-232-NDSC (toll-free outside IL)

SUPPORT AND INFORMATION FOR PARENTS
Compassionate Friends
P.O. Box 3696
Oak Brook, IL 60522
312-990-0010
Support for families over the death of a child

National Sudden Infant Death Syndrome Foundation
822 Professional Place
Suite 104
Landover, MD 20785
301-459-3388
800-221-SIDS (toll-free)
Referrals to local chapters

Postpartum Support International
c/o Jane Honikman
927 N. Kellogg Ave.
Santa Barbara, CA 93111
805-967-7636
Self-help mutual aid group to support mothers with postpartum emotional syndrome

Parents Anonymous
6733 South Sepulveda Blvd.
Suite 270
Los Angeles, CA 90045
Counseling for parents who have or who are tempted to abuse their children (check phone directory for local chapter or write to the above address)

Stepfamily Association of America, Inc.
602 East Joppa Road
Baltimore, MD 21204
301-823-7570
Clearinghouse for all educational materials dealing with stepfamilies

INFORMATION ON HEALTH, SAFETY AND FIRST AID
American Academy of Pediatrics
141 Northwest Point Blvd.
P.O. Box 927
Elk Grove Village, IL 60007
312-228-5005
800-421-0589 (toll-free IL only)
800-433-9016 (toll-free)
Information and referrals

American Red Cross
National Headquarters
17th and D Sts. N.W.
Washington, D.C. 20006
202-737-8300

National Fire Protection Association
Batterymarch Park
Quincy, MA 02269-9101
617-770-3000
Information on fire safety; planning escape routes in your home

National Safety Council
444 N. Michigan Ave.
Chicago, IL 60611
312-527-4800
800-621-7619 (toll-free)
or 800-421-9585 (toll-free)
Publishes material on safe toys and furniture, safety restraints, etc.

National Highway Traffic Safety Administration
U.S. Department of Transportation
400 7th St. N.W.
Washington, D.C. 20590
202-366-0123
800-424-9393 (toll-free outside Washington, D.C. for information about carseats and automotive safety) For local information, contact your state's Office of Highway Safety

U.S. Consumer Product Safety Commission
1750 K St. N.W.
Washington, D.C. 20207
800-638-2772 (toll-free for complaints about faulty items and information on safe ones)

Index

Acknowledgments

Author's acknowledgments:
With thanks as always to my husband, Nicholas. Also to Nancy Ward; Dr Elizabeth Jones and her colleagues at the Surgery in St Margaret's; the staff at Queen Charlotte's Hospital and my son, Michael, for inspiring me even before he was born.
Conran Octopus wish to thank the following:
For advising on text and illustrations:
Greta Balfour, Professional Officer of the Royal College of Midwives.
For her invaluable help with the American edition: Emily Van Ness
For illustrations: Biz Hull, Annabel Milne
For design help: Claire Graham
For taking part in the photography: Olivia James, Sue and Elliot Rosenberg, Dr Sonia Robertson
For back jacket photograph: Guillaume de Faubier/Pix

For their permission to reproduce photographs: 1 Loisjoy Thurston/Bubbles; **2** Claude Gibault/Jerrican; **4** Loisjoy Thurston/Bubbles; **7** Pictor International; **12** CNRI/Science Photo Library; **17** Loisjoy Thurston/Bubbles; **18** Petit Format/Nestlé/Science Photo Library; **21** Christian Moser/Marie Claire; **22** Petit Format/Nestlé/ Science Photo Library; **23** Sally & Richard Greenhill; **25** Sandra Lousada/Susan Griggs Agency; **26** from *A Colour Atlas of Life Before Birth* by Marjorie A. England published by Wolfe Publishing; **33** Jennie Woodcock; **35** Pictor International; **36** Petit Format/Nestlé/Science Photo Library; **37, 49** Sally & Richard Greenhill; **50** Lupe Cunha; **51** Loisjoy Thurston/Bubbles; **52** Petit Format/Nestlé/Science Photo Library; **55** Camera Press; **63** Loisjoy Thurston/Bubbles; **69** Tim Woodcock; **73, 81, 85** Sally & Richard Greenhill; **86** David Sutherland/Tony Stone Photo Library.